THE STERN CARDIOVASCULAR CENTER
A CENTURY OF EXCELLENCE

By Samantha Crespo

PRODUCED BY CITYINK COMPANY

WWW.CITYINK.COM

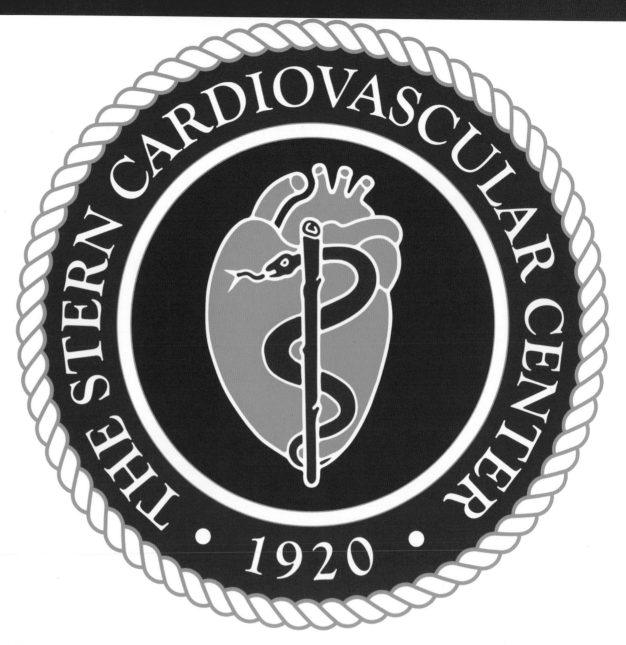

Library of Congress Control Number: 555555555
ISBN-13: 978-0-9741374-4-5
Written by Crespo, Samantha (1977-)
Designed by Towery, Noah (1983-)

Founded by Dr. Neuton S. Stern in 1920, the Stern Cardiovascular Foundation has grown to become the largest cardiovascular group in the tri-state area. Author Samantha Crespo gives a detailed account of how Stern Cardio grew together with the burgeoning medical science of the 20th and 21st centuries. Filled with historical photographs, this volume is a testament to the excellence in care that has become synonymous with the institution.

produced by cityink company
www.cityink.com
Memphis, TN 901-483-2001

Printed in Korea

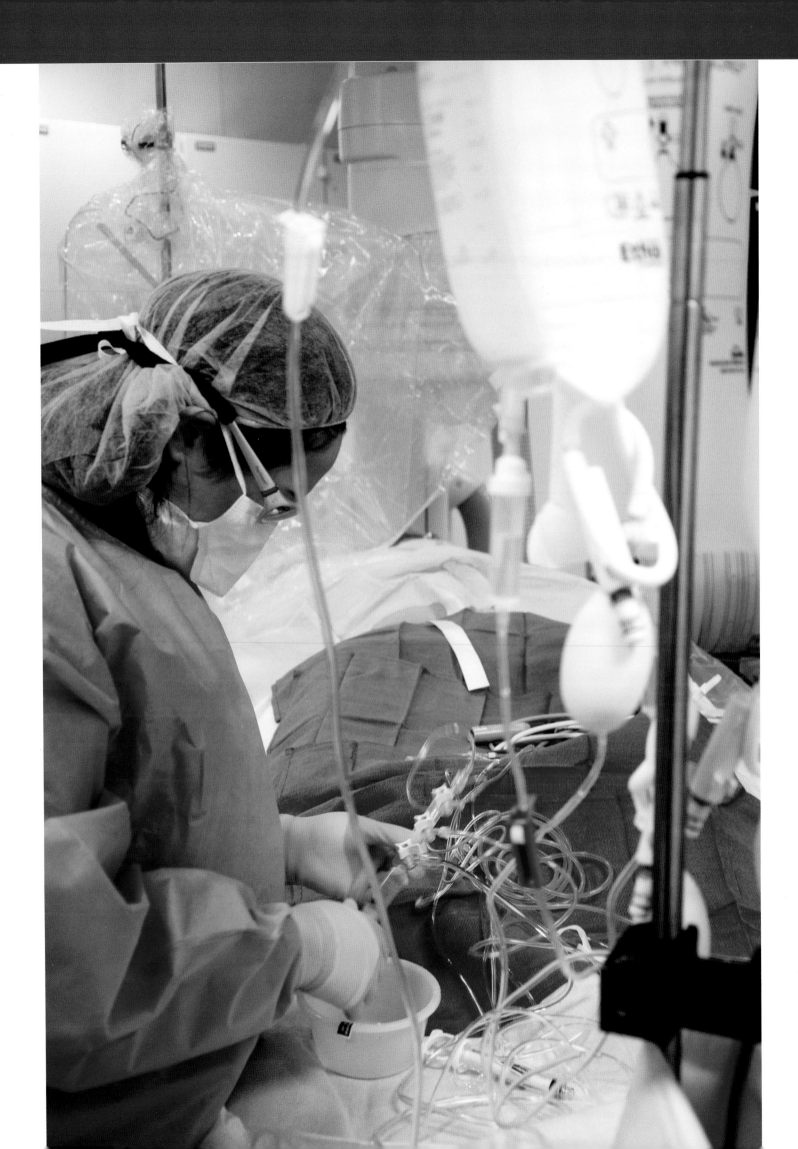

CONTENTS

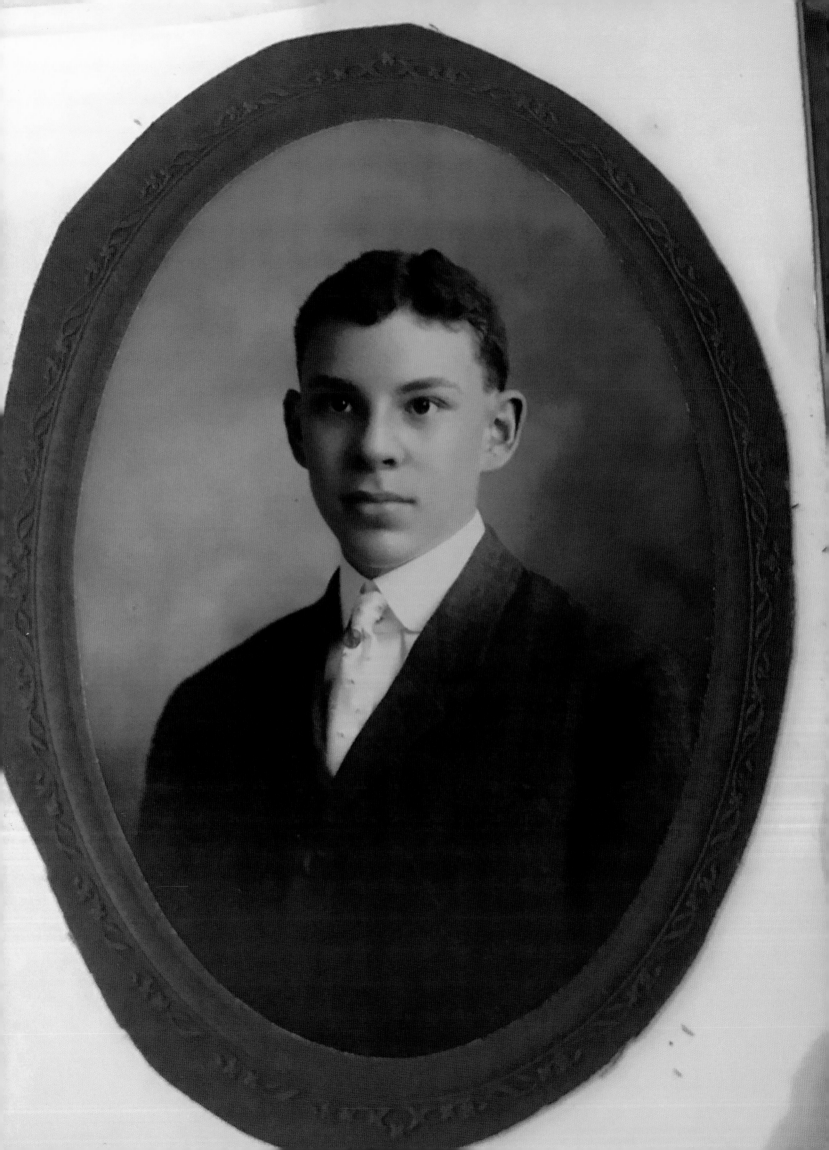

CHAPTER 1 | 1890-1920: NEUTON STERN'S BEGINNINGS

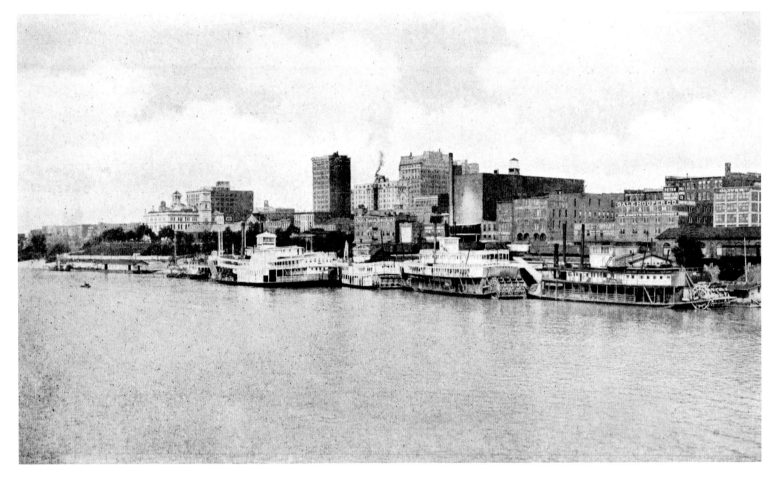

▲ Downtown Memphis in 1921

◀◀ Neuton Stern, age 18

Photo credit: David Stern

IN THE MIDDLE OF THE 19TH CENTURY, A COUPLE IMMIGRATED TO THE U.S. FROM GERMANY. AROUND THE SAME TIME, A FAMILY WAS MAKING ITS NAME—STERN BROS. AUCTIONEERS—IN NEW ORLEANS (BY SMUGGLING SHOES THROUGH CIVIL WAR BLOCKADES, OR SO THE STORIES GO). AS FATE WOULD HAVE IT, THE PARTIES WOULD MEET IN MEMPHIS, TENNESSEE: THE IMMIGRANTS WOULD BECOME THE MATERNAL GRANDPARENTS OF ONE NEUTON SAMUEL STERN; THE NEW ORLEANS CREW WOULD REPRESENT NEUTON'S PATERNAL ROOTS. AS SUSAN EDELMAN AND DAVID STERN, M.D., NEUTON'S GRANDCHILDREN, UNDERSTAND, THE STERN FAMILY WAS INSTALLED IN NEW ORLEANS PRIOR TO THE CIVIL WAR. STILL, THEIR PATERNAL GREAT-GRANDFATHER TRADED THE CRESCENT CITY FOR THE BLUFF CITY, WHERE HE WOULD OPERATE A GENERAL STORE IN THE PINCH DISTRICT.

When Neuton Stern was born on April 9, 1890, his hometown held in its collective memory the loss of its charter—and more than half of its population—due to the yellow fever epidemics of the 1870s. But Neuton's birth coincided with the period of Memphis' rebirth: In 1893, Robert Church Sr. purchased the first bond to help the city recover from bankruptcy, then invested in real estate on and around Beale Street. Here, musicians began sounding the first notes in a sonic legacy that would eventually span the world, and the centuries. Five years later, the grand Orpheum Theatre celebrated its opening night just down the street. By the turn of the 20th century, the city's main industry—

cotton production—demonstrated strong growth. And, of particular interest to the story we'll tell in this book, the city of Memphis began creating policy around public health.

"Memphis conquered her diseases and scrubbed away her filth, and out of the chaotic 1800s there emerged a new city, founded solidly on principles of public health and hygiene."

—Eugene W. Fowinkle, M.D., and Mildred Hicks, excerpted from History of Medicine in Memphis

The Education of Neuton Stern

Though Neuton graduated from Memphis' Central High School, an aunt on his father's side had a different plan in mind. Aunt Frances Stern worked as a nutritionist in Boston, Massachusetts. (The Frances Stern Nutrition Center remains a fixture of the city's Tufts Medical Center today.) Susan Edelman shares a distillation of Aunt Frances' plan: "She felt that her brilliant nephew had not gotten enough education in Memphis, and that he needed another year." David Stern relays a longer version, which his father, Tom Stern, heard from a cousin: "[Aunt Frances] came to visit Memphis. A relative was hiding behind the staircase when there was an intense discussion between Frances and [Neuton's] parents about it being a waste to have such a smart boy work at a factory in Memphis, and her insisting he come to Boston."

Details of this passed-along story match other family lore, according to David. "I always hear that Morris Stern, my great-grand-

father, wanted my grandfather, Neuton, to work in a factory or work in Memphis in a merchant business," David says. Was Frances merely determined to give Neuton what she deemed to be a proper education? Or was she saving her nephew from a career she feared would limit his potential? Perhaps both; perhaps something slightly more strategic: "It was her opinion that Neuton would not be fit for training at Harvard without an additional year of high school," David offers.

Whatever Aunt Frances' true motivation, Neuton went to live with her in Boston, where it is said he attended Boston Latin School for one year before completing Harvard University (1912) and ultimately, Harvard Medical School (1916). As Aunt Frances had suspected, Neuton thrived in the Ivy League ecosystem. "One of my grandfather's Harvard Medical School classmates donated his papers," David notes, one of which revealed a list of grades from the class' final examination. "My grandfather ended up at the top of the class," David says.

An Internship, a World War and an Opportunity

Following his internship at Boston's Massachusetts General Hospital, Neuton Stern enlisted in the U.S. Army Medical Corps. Sources place him at Fort Sill in Oklahoma, where divisions mustered at Camp Doniphan prior to deploying to Europe. Born of necessity in 1917, the camp was an alternately dusty and muddy tent city where tens of thousands of men—including former U.S. President Harry S. Truman—trained for the hardships ahead. The curriculum, as

taught by members of the U.S. Army Medical Department like Neuton, included the new subject of defending oneself against gas warfare.

The lessons of Camp Doniphan weren't all theoretical, however. David Stern discovered an article from the American Laryngological Association entitled "Demonstration of D. Meningitis in the Adenoid Tissue of the Nasopharynx." The article details an epidemic of meningitis at Fort Doniphan between November 1917 and February 1918. "It goes on to talk about what they did and the doctors involved. If you look at the end of the article, after the references, it says, 'We desire to thank 1st Lt. Neuton Stern for the photomicrograph of this case,'" David reads, noting the omission of his grandfather's name from the article proper. "Certainly, he was there. He obviously participated in the research and created the micrograph. But they did not choose to put his name on the paper," David notes, wondering aloud if some combination of Neuton's youth, Jewish heritage, Boston training and "fancy ideas" stigmatized him among the ranks of his new milieu.

Whatever the case, the first lieutenant was met with a different reaction upon deployment "over there." Though the conditions of its conferment are elusive, we know that Neuton Stern returned from Europe with a medal from the French government, presumably for halting an epidemic similar to the one he encountered at Fort Doniphan. In the Spring 1998 newsletter of the Jewish Historical Society of Memphis & the Mid-South, Southern Jewish

▶ Neuton Stern's medal for service in France during the Spanish Flu epidimic of 1919

Photo credit: David Stern

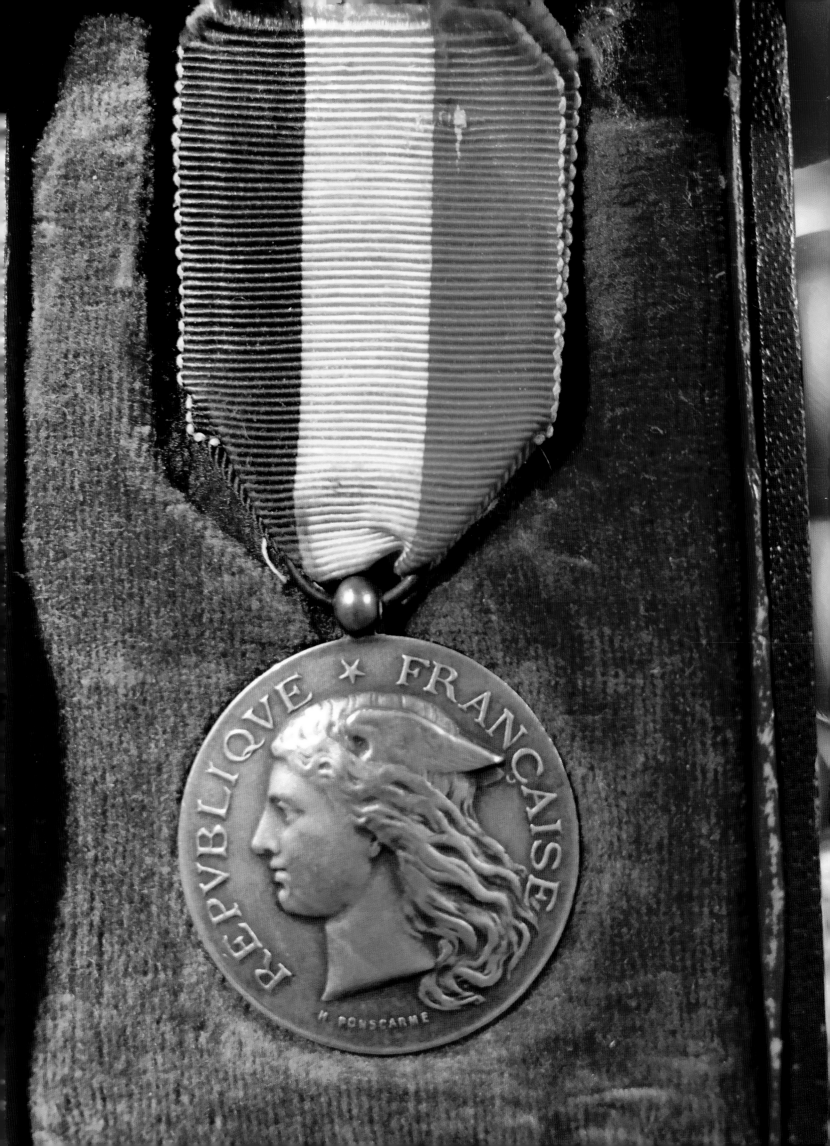

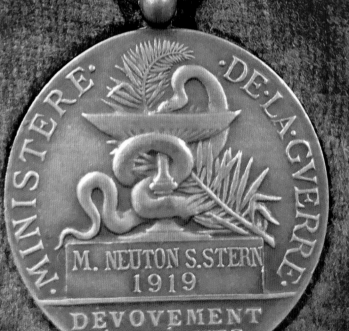

Heritage, the front page featured a spotlight on Dr. and Mrs. Neuton Stern. The article elucidated the conditions under which Neuton received the medal of honor of the French Republic in 1919: "The newly graduated doctor was court-martialed by the U.S. Army for using a vaccine against meningitis, a treatment with which he was familiar before the Army was aware of it." As we now understand, Neuton was exonerated, then decorated, for his life-saving intervention. A synopsis of his service follows, as researched by Tim Harrison, husband of Sharon Harrison, Director of Human Resources and Front Office for Stern Cardiovascular Foundation:

"Neuton Samuel Stern was commissioned a 1st Lieutenant in the Medical Corps, U.S. Army Reserves, on September 7, 1917. He graduated from the U.S. Army Medical School that same year. From September 16 - December 1, 1917, he was assigned to the Medical Officers Training Camp at Fort Benjamin Harrison, Indiana. From December 8, 1917 - July 4, 1918, he was assigned to the Base Hospital at Fort Sill, Oklahoma. He sailed for France aboard the S.S. Empress of Britain on July 14, 1918. On August 9, 1918, he was assigned Assistant to the Chief Purchasing Officer, Medical Department, in Paris, France, and remained in that position until his discharge on October 11, 1919, in France."

The European post would hold a golden opportunity for Neuton: access to the London laboratory of Sir Thomas Lewis.

MASTERING THE ELECTROCARDIOGRAPH

"The time is at hand, if not already come, when an examination of the heart is incomplete if this new method is neglected. —Sir Thomas Lewis, a pioneer of modern cardiology

It was Neuton Stern's interest in the human heart that would lead him to Sir Thomas Lewis. David Stern imagines how compelling the opportunity would have been for his grandfather. At the time, the understanding "that there were electrical pulses in the heart, and that those pulses might tell you something about the structure or function of the heart, was a pretty interesting leap," David explains. Indeed: As intellectuals attempted to understand the still-fresh medical hypothesis, citizens at-large grappled with the very concept of electricity. (It wasn't until 1925 that even half of U.S. homes would be equipped with electric power.) Sir Thomas Lewis worked at the intersection of these newfangled ideas, and Neuton arranged to be decommissioned from the Army in order to study with him.

Lewis had been a student of Willem Einthoven, who had himself studied under Augustus Waller, the British physiologist who recorded the first human electrocardiogram in 1887. Einthoven improved on Waller's design, producing in 1901 a string galvanometer that used three leads and coining the term 'electrocardiogram'—the invention of which earned him the 1924 Nobel Prize in physiology and medicine. In his Nobel lecture, Einthoven credited Lewis, saying, "It is my conviction that the general interest in the

ECG would certainly not be so high nowadays if we had to do without his work, and I doubt whether without his valuable contribution I should have the privilege of standing before you today."

From 1908 through 1920, Lewis, installed at University College Hospital in London, pushed the capabilities of the new technology to become a leader in the burgeoning field. As the first person to acquire an electrocardiogram for clinical research, Lewis focused on cardiac arrhythmias, using the ECG to discover that irregular heartbeat was a result of atrial fibrillation. His personal approach—augmenting clinical practice with laboratory research and emerging technology—exemplified a greater shift occurring in medicine at the time. It also attracted a new generation of heart specialists from Britain and America who came to observe and conduct their own research under Lewis' tutelage.

Thus, Neuton's stint in Lewis' lab was spent in good company. He was joined by two friends: Samuel A. Levine and Paul Dudley White. Sam Levine was a medical school classmate of Neuton's who would later lend his name to Levine's Sign, a clenched fist held over the chest to indicate ischemic chest pain. As for Paul Dudley White, let's hear from Frank McGrew, M.D., who would practice with Neuton's son, Tom, more than 50 years later.

When Frank developed an interest in the history of the practice he joined in 1976, he spoke to Neuton's widow, Beatrice "Bea" Stern. "She told me several things about Neuton. One of his friends

◀ Neuton Stern's medal for service in France during the Spanish Flu epidimic of 1919

Photo credit: David Stern

from his school days—they were also in the Army together—was Paul Dudley White. When the war was over, they both worked with Sir Thomas Lewis before coming back to the states," Frank relays. White went on to become a founder of the American Heart Association, to play a major role in establishing the National Institutes of Health and the Framingham Heart Study, and to serve as U.S. President Dwight D. Eisenhower's cardiologist. Widely regarded as the founder of preventive cardiology, "White was the first cardiologist whose name was a household word," Frank explains.

While the daily trials and triumphs of Lewis' lab have largely been lost to history, we're treated to one glimpse passed down from Neuton to Tom to David, who tells it like this: "They used to make EKGs on a big drum that they wrapped a piece of smoked paper around. A needle would be touching the smoked paper as the drum would go around in a circle and the needle would scratch the dark smoke off of the paper. These were called smoke-drum tracings."

During his time in London, Neuton also spent a half-day of each week with Sir James Mackenzie, a Scottish cardiologist who moved his medical practice to London to help further the study of cardiac arrhythmias. Like Lewis, Mackenzie's focus was broader than the technology. The two represented a relatively novel notion at the time: For the best chance of a positive outcome, physicians should consider a patient's concerns through the lens of disordered function.

Certainly, Neuton Stern was influenced by the approach modeled by Lewis and Mackenzie when it came to collecting patient histories and conducting physical examinations. But beyond the daily routine of patient visits, the big picture—merging clinical practice with research and technology—would make the greatest impact on young Neuton Stern.

Neuton Stern.
Photos thanks to David Stern.

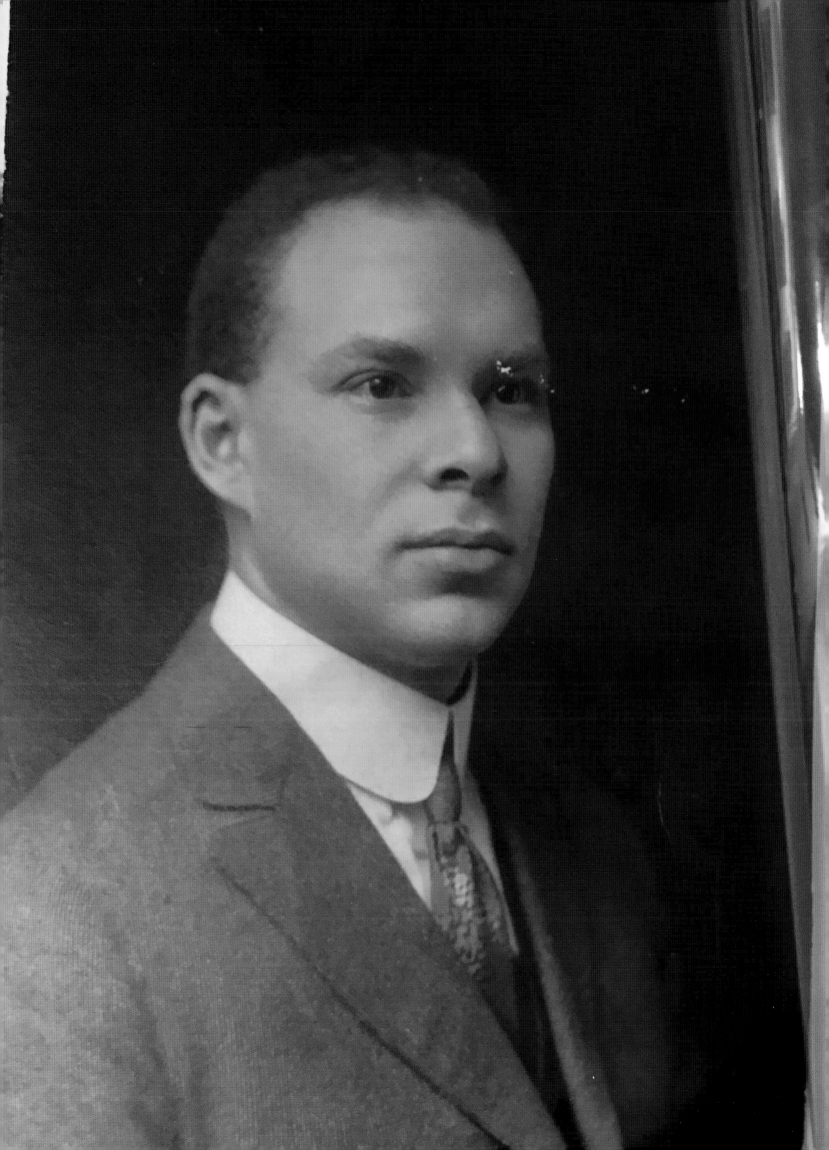

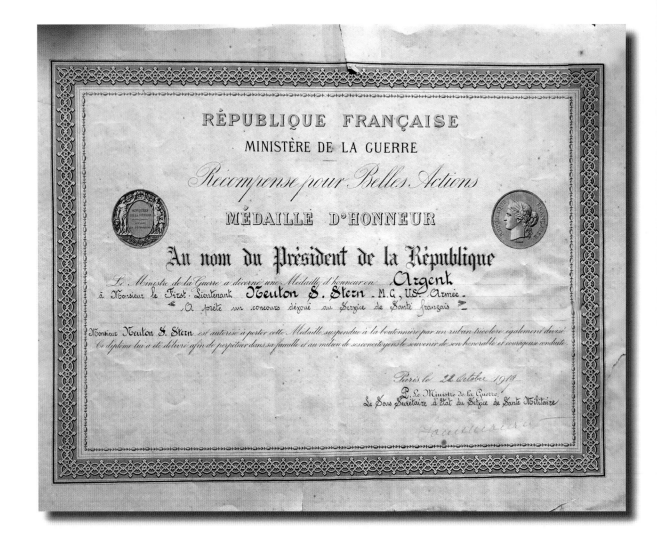

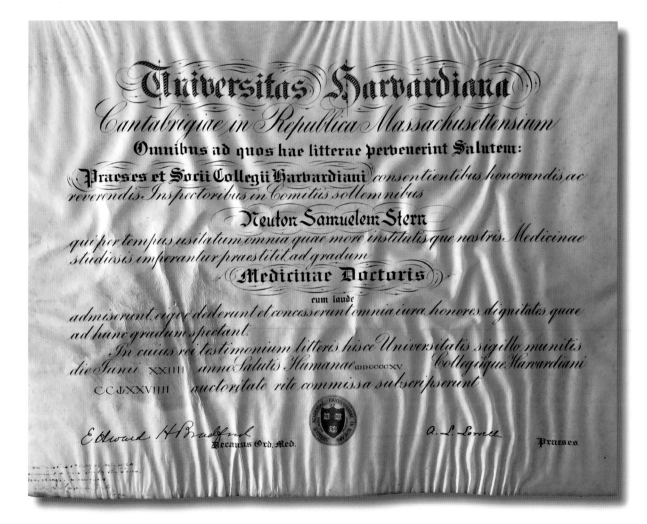

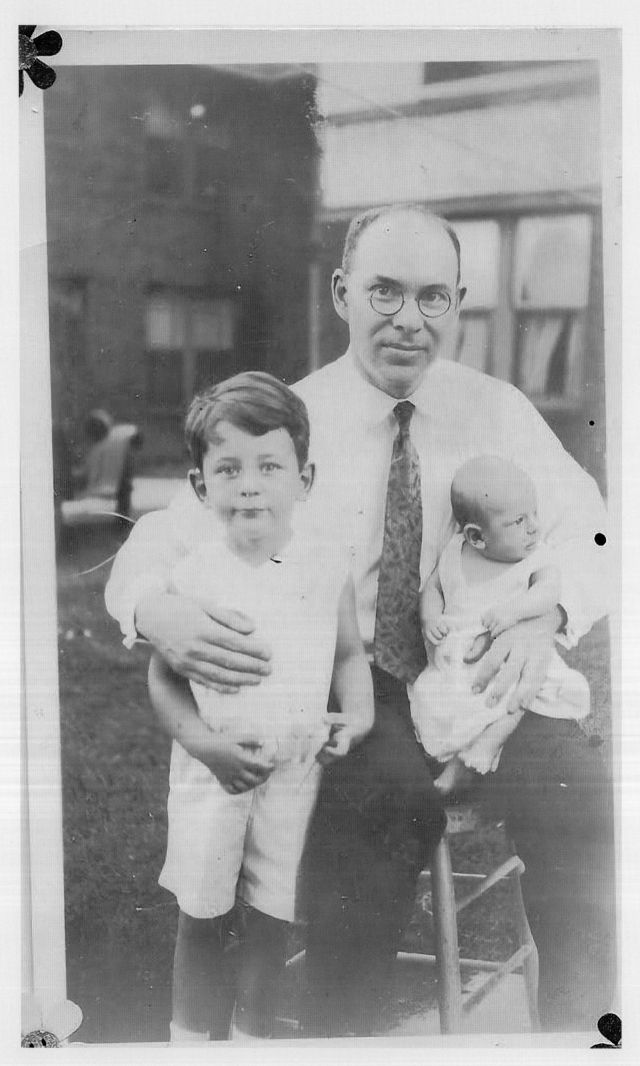

Stern Cardiovascular Foundation

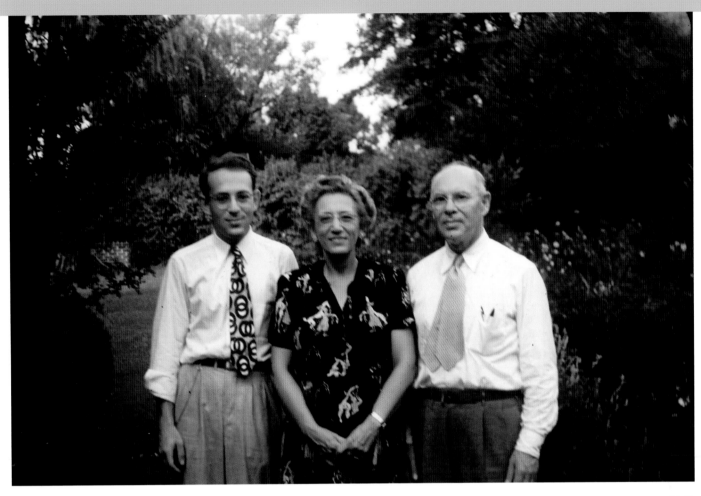

◀▲ The Stern family
photo credit: David Stern.

AFTER LOGGING A YEAR IN LEWIS' LAB, NEUTON PREPARED FOR A HOMECOM-ING—AND A DECISION. IT WAS TIME TO HANG UP HIS SHINGLE, SO TO SPEAK, BUT WHERE? THERE WAS AN INVITATION TO RETURN TO MASSACHUSETTS GENERAL AND JOIN THE FACULTY, BUT "HE FELT THAT MEMPHIS WAS IN NEED OF HIGH-QUAL-ITY MEDICAL CARE AND HIGHLY TRAINED PHYSICIANS," SAYS SUSAN EDELMAN.

With the announcement of Neuton's decision, David Stern notes, Aunt Frances "won the battle but lost the war." While she had managed to shepherd her nephew through the Boston-based training that would enable him to write his own ticket anywhere, "Neuton was deeply committed to coming back to Memphis," David says. The pull of the nuclear family seems to have been a factor as well.

NAVIGATING MEMPHIS' MEDICAL LANDSCAPE

By the time Neuton returned to his hometown in 1920, the city was busy responding to the recommendations of a health department survey conducted by Paul Preble, former Assistant Surgeon for the U.S. Public Health Service. Preble recommended the appointment of a full-time superintendent for the city's health department

and a complete departmental re-organization. Once the establishment of a Chair of Public Health at the University of Tennessee Medical School made the former possible, the city set about the latter. Within one year, a full-time director for communicable disease control was appointed, a "sanitary engineer" initiated a malaria control program and a division of dental hygiene was organized (one of the first free dental clinics in the country to be operated by a health department)—followed by a department of maternal and child hygiene. Amid the flurry of organizational changes, Memphis saw its first use of epidemiological case records and chronological charts. Even before 1920, standards were improving: "At the close of World War I, organization of schools of public health for training health officers created a new era in public health and provided a stimulus for the protection of personal health" (Stewart, Black & Hicks, 1971).

One might surmise, then, that Neuton Stern—Harvard Medical School standout, decorated veteran, student of the venerated Sir Thomas Lewis, ambitious young internist—would be enthusiastically welcomed by his colleagues in a modernizing Memphis.

Yet, in this era, influences such as folksy wisdom, a commitment to the status quo and ego could cast doubt on science. The city's Superintendent of Health appointed in 1927, L. M. Graves, endorsed eating apples for health and refraining from "kissing your girl if you want to escape the flu"— while simultaneously urging students to "protect their lives against the mad rush of the 'jazz age.'" It was into this context—of shifting cultural values and the nascence of modern medicine—that Neuton Stern, M.D., presented a paper on the electrocardiograph, and the machine itself. The machine had been adapted for commercial use a scant decade prior.

In a retrospective written by Neuton's son, Thomas, we learn how the presentation was received:

"Soon after [his] arrival [in Memphis], he gave a paper at a meeting of the Medical Society on the electrograph. Giving such papers was the standard way for young doctors to become known in the community. After he finished, one of the senior physicians stood up to comment; he announced that any doctor who needed such a machine to help him had no business calling himself a doctor. This sentiment was seconded by another of the medical notables of the time. Needless to say, they both used the EKG later in their lives." — Thomas Stern, M.D., excerpted from "Memphis Cardiology in Retrospect"

Thus, Neuton Stern set up practice as an internist with a special interest in the heart—and the first electrocardiograph in the Southern U.S. According to Beatrice Stern, Neuton's practice was the only heart center at the time between Chicago and New Orleans.

THE DAWN OF A GOLDEN AGE

Despite some evidence to the contrary, this was a new age in medicine—the dawn of what some call the "golden age." Beyond the innovation of new technologies, consider the advancements in education, regulation and organization that occurred in the years adjacent to Neuton's training:

In 1904, the American Medical Association (AMA) formed the Council on Medical Education to establish licensure standards for physicians.

In the first decade of the 20th century, AMA membership increased from 8,000 to 70,000.

Culturally, American acceptance of medicine as a science led to the emergence of hospitals as credible centers for treatment.

The American College of Surgeons was founded in 1913 as the first body to accredit hospitals.

By the 1920s and the start of Neuton Stern's professional practice, sub-specialties began to take shape. While cardiology was beginning to be recognized as a sub-specialty, internists and university centers were more likely to declare the heart as a special interest, rather than declare themselves as cardiologists and cardiology centers. "People like Neuton and Sam Levine became cardiologists before there were cardiologists," David Stern says. Indeed, Neuton is considered to be the first cardiologist to practice in the Southern U.S. Still, Neuton would further distinguish himself in the field of internal medicine, this time by sitting for the examination of the newly formed American Board of Internal Medicine (ABIM).

Responding to the public call for physicians to follow more uniform standards, ABIM was founded in 1936. Today, more than 200,000 internists have been certified, demonstrating the clinical judgment, skills and attitude required to deliver excellent patient care. Neuton Stern, with about a dozen cohorts, constituted the second group of individuals ever to achieve certification by the physician-led, non-profit organization for the independent evaluation of physicians.

Of the markers of her grandfather's and father's prodigious careers, Susan Edelman notes that the family has always strived to display mementos in their proper places. For this reason, Neuton Stern's ABIM certificate,

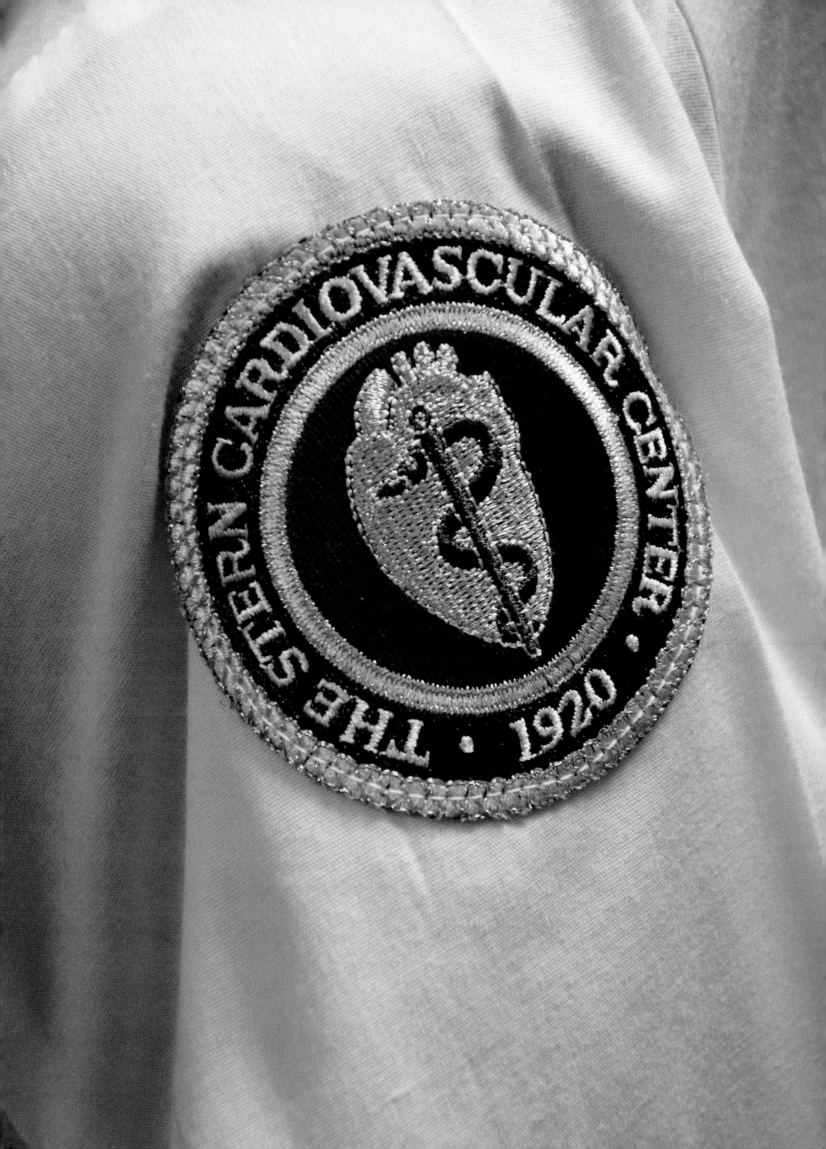

dated July 1, 1937, now hangs in the organization's Philadelphia office. E-mail correspondence to David Stern from Richard J. Baron, current President and CEO of the American Board of Internal Medicine and the ABIM Foundation, notes:

"... wanted you to see what we did with your [grandfather's] certificate: one photo shows how it was framed, with the bio; the other photo is where we placed it, which is to say, right next to the front door ... Thanks so much for sharing it. We are really proud to have it and be able to display it in such a place of honor!"

What's more, ABIM recently redesigned its certificate to more closely resemble those issued in the 1930s. Neuton Stern's certificate served as a visual reference for the new design. A photograph of his certificate, along with a synopsis of his professional journey, are now included in the welcome kit that ABIM sends to 30,000 newly certified physicians annually. "These are physicians who have just passed their initial board certification exam, and we thought sharing some of Neuton's story would serve as an inspiration to them as they begin their careers," notes John Held, Director of Communications and Brand Management for ABIM.

Day-to-Day Operations

Tributes such as the ABIM certificate document major points in the developing narrative of Neuton Stern. But what of the quotidien? David Stern keeps his grandfather's original nameplate, which reads: Neuton Stern, Internal Medicine and Cardiology. Susan Edelman recalls stories of Depression-era patients leaving eggs or baskets of fruits and vegetables at her grandparents' door as payment for care. "They wouldn't turn anybody away," she explains. For all of its proven benefits, the EKG continued to confound some folks. You might even sympathize, considering what Beatrice Stern told Frank McGrew: The machine took up an entire room and was expensive to fix. When it broke down, they had to go to the bank to borrow money, as the parts had to be ordered from Europe. And in 1933, Neuton hired one of his earliest employees. After graduating from Mississippi College for Women with a four-year degree in laboratory technology, Mildred Pepper Chambers answered an ad placed by Neuton to help staff his practice. (Mildred would work for the practice for an additional 40-odd years, continuing to conduct her blood analyses manually, the method in which she was trained.)

And what of the stigma that may or may not have kept Neuton's name off of the paper regarding the epidemic at Camp Doniphan? In 1968, Beatrice and Neuton Stern would participate in an oral history project conducted by Dr. Berkley Kalin of Memphis State University, now the University of Memphis. During those interviews, Kalin asked Neuton about a stalled effort to build a Jewish hospital in Memphis in the 1920s. Neuton's response:

"We would, of course, have supported it if it had been built, but we felt that the relationships with the doctors in Memphis—the other doctors—were so good and the relationships with the hospitals of the Jewish doctors were so good that we hesitated by taking a step in the direction of cutting ourselves off to disturb this very friendly and cordial relationship among the medical profession."

When Kalin followed up to establish whether this kind of collaboration was unique to Memphis, Neuton added:

"In old sections of the country—in the East, for instance—many of the hospitals were closed, constantly, and nobody could practice there except the members of the staff. Now, in the city of Memphis all the hospitals were developed with an open staff—that is, men who are ... of good reputation and members of the Medical Society could be voted upon by the different boards and allowed to practice in those hospitals."

As the interview continued, Beatrice recounted a conversation with a Dr. Fineshriber in the 1930s. The doctor asked, "Do you have any non-Jewish patients?" The transcript of Beatrice's response continues as follows:

"And Neuton said, 'Indeed I do. I would say that it is at least 75 per cent non-Jewish and 25 per cent Jewish.' Dr. Fineshriber expressed amazement, and said this was simply unbelievable. He said that [this] would not happen, and does not happen, in one of the big Eastern cities unless you just happen to be the most famous man in your field."

When Kalin noted that these stories, taken together, spoke well for integration, Neuton clarified: "[They] speak well for integration of Jewish doctors and for the whole general community in their acceptance."

Establishing a Family

The same oral history interview transcripts feature the following recollection from Beatrice Stern:

"When I came back here for the first time to Memphis, about 1917 or '18, there were no boys here to go out with. They were all in service."

Neuton, as we know, was among them, one of approximately 9,000 Memphis-area men who served in World War I. When the boys returned, a social custom helped them "reacclimate." As Susan Edelman explains, "Jewish families from St. Louis to New Orleans, Kansas City to Chattanooga would have house parties where young Jewish people could meet each other. My own parents met at a house party like that."

Considering this, does it seem so far-fetched that Neuton met Beatrice Wolf when he breezed into a house party on a slide—set up just for the occasion—and landed at her feet?

We may never definitively know what led to Neuton and Bea's first meeting, but records help piece together what came next: marriage in 1924; a son, Thomas N., born on April 22, 1926 and named for Sir Thomas Lewis; a home, built in 1928, at 684 Center Drive in Memphis' leafy Hein Park neighborhood. As Susan shares, her father "mostly grew up there. He could hear lions roaring in the morning [from nearby Memphis Zoo]. He went to Snowden School, then Central High School."

Mentoring and Organizing

Perhaps inspired by the opportunity he had been afforded at the onset of his career, Neuton Stern began offering work to young internists in the 1940s. At the same time, Memphis was committing to the Allied war effort. Between 1940 and 1943, the city built a naval air station; kicked defense plants, depots and an armory into gear; sent native son Luke Weathers over Europe in a B-24 bomber called The Spirit of Beale Street and inspired the naming of the B-17 Memphis Belle, thanks to local sweetheart Margaret Polk.

In time, many of the internists Neuton employed were called to answer a higher duty: serving in the United States Armed Forces. That didn't stop Neuton from recruiting some of them right back following the war's close. Daniel A. Brody, M.D., was one such recruit. Under the mentorship of Neuton Stern, Brody cultivated an interest in electrocardiography, eventually becoming a professor of medicine and Chief of the Section of Cardiovascular Diseases at the University of Tennessee College of Medicine. Brody went on to develop digital computer applications within his area of interest, ultimately earning a Research Career Award from the National Institutes of Health in 1962 and defining the Brody Effect, relating the electrical resistivity of intracardiac blood to the surrounding tissues. Like Lewis, Mackenzie and Stern before him, Brody devoted time to mentoring the next generation, advancing the field of theoretical electrocardiography.

Despite, or perhaps because of, the global upheaval of the 1940s,

local and national healthcare grew more organized throughout the decade. In 1949, for example, the American College of Cardiology was founded in New York City, paving the way for cardiology to fully distinguish itself as a sub-specialty of internal medicine. For Neuton, the changes must have been welcome; over the course of his career, he organized and led several initiatives of his own. Among them: becoming Tennessee's first diplomate of the National Board of Medical Examiners; founding and presiding over the Memphis Academy of Medicine, an association of local internists; authoring the Memphis Medical Journal; establishing the Memphis Heart Association (1948) and serving as the group's president—all while leading what would soon become a growing practice.

Memphis: A Hub for Innovation

In bringing innovation to his hometown, you could say that Neuton Stern was just doing his duty as a Memphian. Certainly, the city is synonymous with change-making: Abe Plough parlayed a $125 investment into one of the world's largest pharmaceutical companies. Elvis Presley and Sam Phillips ignited the rock 'n' roll revolution; Jim and Estelle Axton kindled the soul music explosion. Kemmons Wilson disrupted the motel industry, creating the standard for hotels worldwide. Against all odds, Danny Thomas opened St. Jude Children's Research Hospital. And a student named Fred Smith wrote a term paper exploring the concept of reliable overnight delivery service.

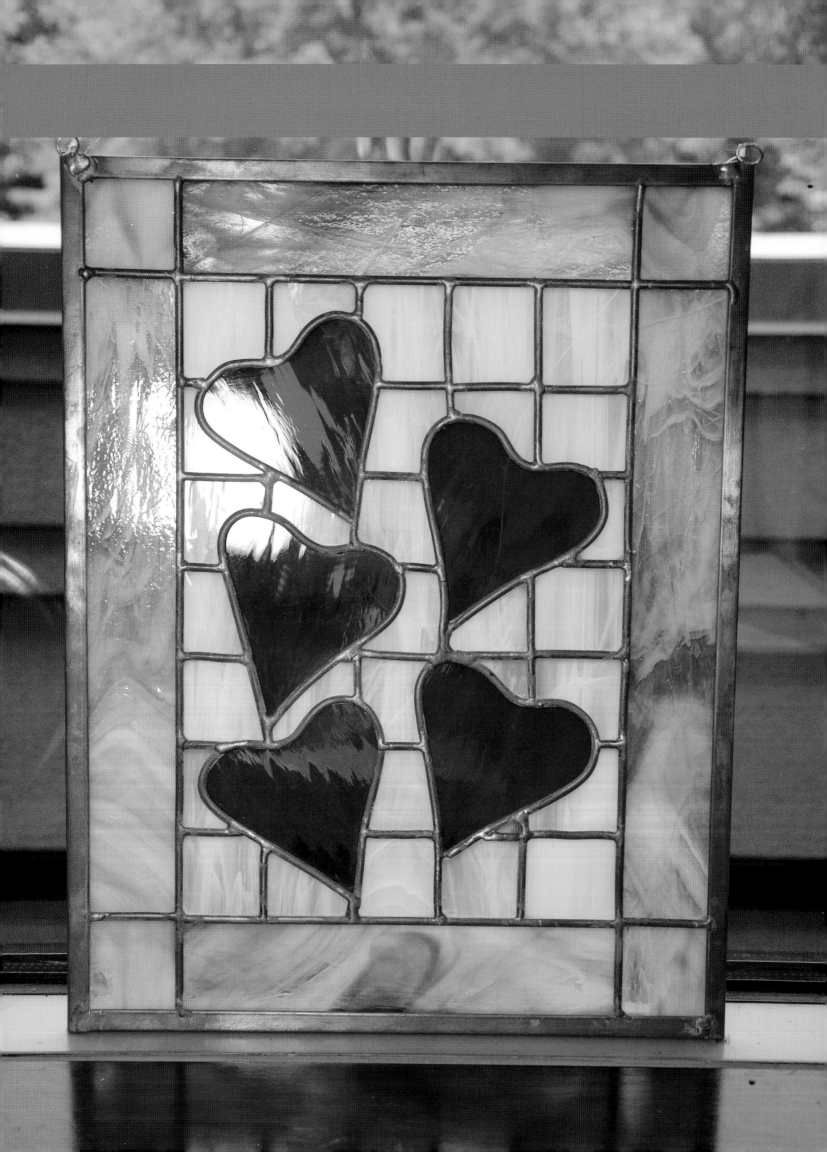

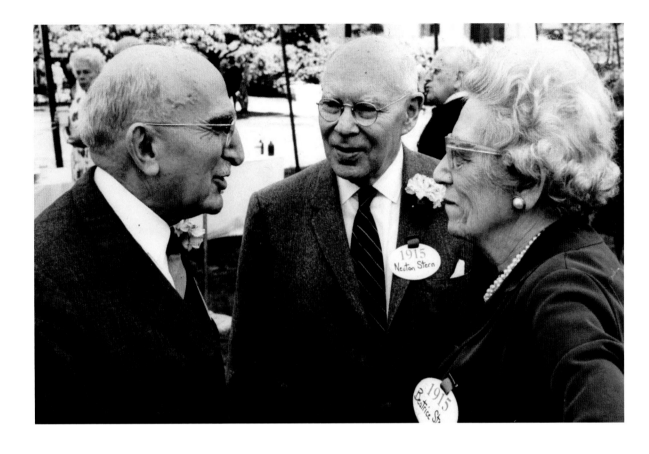

◀ Bea and Neuton Stern.
photo courtesy of David Stern.

◀◀ Stained glass at the clinic.
Photo by Stephanie Norwood.

WHILE THE 1940S REPRESENTED A GATHERING TIME FOR THE FIELD OF CAR-DIOLOGY, THE DECADE ENDED WITH A VERY PERSONAL GATHERING AMONG THE STERN FAMILY. IN 1949, NEUTON STERN SUFFERED HIS FIRST MYOCAR-DIAL INFARCTION. HIS SON THOMAS (TOM) HAD JUST WRAPPED AN INTERNSHIP AND WAS EMBARKING ON A THREE-YEAR RESIDENCY PROGRAM IN INTERNAL MEDICINE. IT SEEMED LIKE AN APT TIME FOR THE YOUNGER STERN TO RETURN TO MEMPHIS.

Like his father, Tom graduated from Memphis' Central High School and Harvard University. Afterward, he completed a hybrid program between the University of Tennessee College of Medicine and Washington University School of Medicine in St. Louis. "He was thinking about going to work at the university—teaching and being more involved in academia at the University of Tennessee—instead of working with my grandfather," David Stern reveals.

Neuton's heart attack changed Tom's mind. "He felt like he had to go take care of my grandfather's patients; he felt an obligation to the patients and to the practice," David explains.

Tom's resolve calls to mind Neuton's own decision to return to Memphis some 30 years earlier. Father and son shared that commitment to family and community, and now they shared a practice, too. Interrupted only by his U.S. Army service, as a captain in Korea in 1953 and 1954, Tom described practicing medicine alongside his father as "a long and wonderful relationship." As David remembers, "My father adored his father and loved practicing with him every day."

THE FIRST CATH LAB

The Sterns also shared a commitment to staying at the forefront of their advancing specialty. In 1950, John Pervis Milnor Jr., M.D.—a fellow Memphian and medical resident with Harvard Services at

Boston City Hospital—was appointed Chief of Medical Services and Director of Internal Medicine Education for Memphis' Baptist Memorial Hospital. Prior to accepting the appointment, Milnor, a National Institutes of Health Research Fellow in Cardiology, established Tulane University School of Medicine's cardiac catheterization program. If such a program could be piloted in New Orleans, why not Memphis? By 1951, John Pervis Milnor Jr. and Tom Stern were collaborating on what Tom characterized as a "very primitive" cardiac catheterization laboratory at Memphis' John Gaston Hospital.

AS TOM DOCUMENTED IN HIS RETROSPECTIVE:

"We used the fluoroscope in the medical outpatient clinic. Venous pressures, including central venous pressures, were recorded on a very cumbersome instrument developed by Dr. George Burch in New Orleans. In 1952, we exercised patients using the master two-step test. Following instructions in one of the heart journals, I devised a very simple telemetry unit using a couple of capacitors and a 25-cent piece. This allowed us to transmit the EKG from the walking patient to the recorder without the necessity of wires."

Within one year, Tom was deployed abroad. But serendipity struck. Toward the end of his service, Tom spent time observing in the laboratory of André F. Cournand. Cournand, pulmonary physiologist and professor of medicine at Columbia University, led the cardiopulmonary lab at Bellevue Hospital in New York City. His exploration of the diagnostic potential of cardiac catheterization, along with collaborators Werner Forssman and Dickinson W. Richards, earned the trio the 1956 Nobel Prize in Physiology or Medicine. Incidentally, Cournand had, as Tom recounted, "a young fellow working with him at the time named Eugene Braunwald." In time, that young fellow would become one of the preeminent practitioners of modern cardiology.

Returned to Memphis, Tom drew on his observations of Cournand's laboratory to refine the setup at Gaston, using the hospital's X-ray department. He was unable to persuade Memphis' Baptist Memorial Hospital to establish a laboratory of its own, but that didn't stop him from performing cardiac catheterizations on-site. Rather, he fashioned an X-ray room inside his and father's office on the hospital's second floor. In the history he penned, "Memphis Cardiology in Retrospect," Tom documented the following:

"Our X-ray room was only six or seven feet wide. Although adequately long, there was hardly room for the patient, me and a few instruments. By that time, we had strain gauges. I converted an old EKG machine into a recorder, and it was actually stationed a couple of feet away in the adjoining dark room. The setup was crude but effective. We did many successful right heart catheterizations leading frequently to surgery."

Though Nancy Hardin was hired as Neuton's assistant in 1954 while Tom was still enlisted, she lent support to Tom as soon as he joined the practice. This included assisting with catheterizations. "Dr. Tom would have the cath in place and I would snap the pictures with the X-ray machine and develop them," Nancy describes.

DIY DIAGNOSTICS

Even while performing the new-generation catheterization procedure, Tom Stern was thinking of further opportunities to advance patient diagnostics. "We always tried to stay in the forefront of technology," he emphasized in his retrospective, recounting other examples from his and his father's practice throughout the 1950s:

While Isaac Starr, M.D., who had developed the first viable ballistocardiography instrument, floated patients on an air mattress resting on a bed of mercury, the Sterns adopted their own approach to studying the motion of the body imparted by the heartbeat. As Tom explained:

"We . . . had an instrument that would approximate the results. Vectorcardiograms could always be calculated from the regular leads but for several years we used an instrument which would integrate the information for us. This didn't turn out to be very useful except in the case of inferior infarction; the VCG would help us decide whether an inferior Q [wave] was positional or due to an infarct.

When the only way to measure thyroid function was to measure a patient's basal metabolic rate, Neuton and Tom "acquired a small instrument that would measure the speed of the ankle jerk reflex, helping greatly in the diagnosis of hyperthyroidism and hypothyroidism," according to Tom's retrospective.

"We measured glucose, BUN and creatinine in the office, cooking the reagents with serum and measuring the developed color on an optical color imager then in a small unit to measure the color intensity. I had worked with Dr. Richard Overman during my residency developing normals for potassium using the newly developed flame photometer but we decided to send electrolyte studies out as the flame instrument was somewhat cumbersome to use at the time," Tom added.

MID-CENTURY THERAPIES AND TREATMENTS

For all of the progress in diagnostics that Neuton and Tom Stern were able to advance, 1950s-era therapeutics were limited. Tom noted the following available therapies in his retrospective:

Digitalis

Quinidine

Procainamide

Nitroglycerin

Pentaerythritol tetranitrate ("There was a dispute about its effectiveness," Tom recalled, but he was convinced, adding: "I knew early on that it was effective, as it relieved some of my patients with angina who had been tried on several of the other suggested drugs. I was sure that this was not [a] placebo effect.")

Mercurials ("The only diuretics available," Tom noted, recounting: "At the city hospital, we had a long line of patients coming in two or three times a week for their injections. I think they probably lost as much ground making the trip in and going home as they did from receiving the mercu hydrin.

Patients also came into our office for their intravenous mercurials. We felt these were more effective than intramuscular.")

Hydrochlorothiazide ("... Available both as a diuretic and [as] an antihypertensive," Tom clarified, adding, "It is, of course, a weak diuretic, but it was better than nothing.")

If the drug therapies available to cardiac patients in the 1950s were limited—and limiting, according to Tom's observations on the administration of mercurials—the treatments were even moreso. Consider how Tom frames a patient's prospects in his retrospective:

"... If the patient had a lot of money, severe hypertension and a great deal of dedication, he could be shipped off to the Rice House at Duke where he would be put on a diet consisting completely of rice for a few weeks. Fruits and vegetables would slowly be added. The treatment was effective but the patients had to be masochists to put up with it."

For acute myocardial infarction, physicians practicing in the 1950s were primarily limited to providing support, a step beyond the standard procedure of the previous decade: prescribing prolonged bed rest. Yet, the Drs. Stern maximized outcomes by adopting a unique approach: delivering highly personalized patient care and innovating that delivery by challenging norms, relentlessly researching and keeping current with new technology. Again, from Tom's retrospective:

"I carried a tank of oxygen in the trunk of my car and an EKG machine. When a patient who

lived in Memphis called with chest pain, I would speed out to their home, take an EKG, start some oxygen and give an injection of intravenous morphine. Usually, I would give intravenous aminophylline ... Once the patient got to the hospital, they were placed in an oxygen tent ... Some patients were given heparin. Coumadin came into frequent usage in the '50s and was given routinely.

"In the early '50s, Dr. Sam Levine, a classmate and close friend of Neuton Stern's, suggested chair rest during the convalescence. However, he recruited four orderlies to pick patients up out of bed and put them in an armchair. We went a little bit further and allowed the patient to get up by themselves with extended periods of chair rest as tolerated.

"Further, Neuton Stern had decided from his reading in the literature that scars were quite strong at two weeks, and there was no necessity to keep a patient in bed and [restrict] activity any longer. We, therefore, only kept our patients in the hospital two weeks as opposed to the otherwise universal six weeks, and we started them on ambulation right away."

To supplement Tom's written record, Nancy Hardin shares her memories of assisting Neuton in the mid-1950s:

"He would put you in the hospital if it looked like you had, or were maybe going to have, a heart attack. Two weeks complete bed rest: He didn't want you to move a muscle until he could get you on nitroglycerin or whatever you needed. Since indigestion, acid reflux, ulcers [and other ailments] can bring on the same symptoms as a heart attack, he made sure.

It took him two to three weeks to make his final diagnosis. If it wasn't a heart attack, he'd tell the patient what they needed to do for the other problems."

And if it was a heart attack?

"I'd go on rounds with him and hear him talk to patients about how they would have to change their lifestyle. They had to eat right and he told them they had to rest every day: get their minds off of their jobs, whatever their way of relaxing. If their pattern was the same when they came back to see him, he told them to get another doctor. He had complete success because his patients had to change their lifestyle. He treated you to get you well," Nancy asserts.

According to Nancy, Neuton's approach to office visits was as careful as his protocol in-hospital. "It took him several visits to give a diagnosis. He went strictly by the stethoscope, the echocardiogram, the X-ray machine and what patients were telling him," she remembers.

A Glimpse into the Office

Whereas Tom Stern's retrospective connects modern-day readers to an otherwise distant period in cardiology, the reflections of Nancy Hardin paint a picture of day-to-day operations inside the Stern clinic—circa 1954.

Nancy came to the clinic at the age of 22 from Memphis' John Gaston Hospital, where she had helped to open a cancer clinic. In addition to assisting with cancer screenings, she trained with a variety of doctors and across disciplines, logging time from the biopsy lab to the autopsy lab. The experience prepared her for her work, and for the additional training she would receive, with Neuton and Tom Stern.

Some of Nancy's tasks required less technical skill than humanity. Her first order of the day: Stop en route to the office to buy a cookie—any variety. Nancy's second assignment was to meet "Dr. Neuton" at his car in order to accompany him into the office, while carrying the doctor's medical bag for him. "They had me do that out of consideration. Neuton was of an age and having spasmodic attacks with his heart. The family told Mildred, our lab supervisor, to always make sure that somebody met him there," Nancy explains. Finally, in a break each afternoon, Nancy was to deliver the cookie she had purchased that morning, along with a glass of milk, on a tray to "Dr. Stern's room." She describes it as a small room in the office furnished with a bed and nightstand—just right for Neuton's afternoon rest. When Tom Stern joined his father at the practice, Nancy remembers two things: "Tom walked his own self to the office, and he had the same disposition his dad did with his employees—just like you were his family. They were the same way with their patients. I don't know anything but the Sterns' humility, kindness and graciousness."

When it came to technical training, Nancy started with "cardiograms, bloodwork . . . everything to work patients up," she describes. Mildred Pepper Chambers was her primary trainer, with the hope that Nancy would assume Mildred's ancillary duties and enable Mildred to focus on the lab. Even so, Nancy remembers Mildred training her to "read blood" using a microscope and drawing blood from a patient when Nancy couldn't quite get the hang of it. If you had taken roll at the office around this time, you'd find:

Two Doctors Stern

One lab supervisor (Mildred Pepper Chambers)

One assistant (Nancy, who handled everything from supporting cutting-edge catheterizations to filing to ensuring that Neuton Stern got his afternoon rest)

One receptionist, who could double as a transcriptionist (nicknamed "Tweaky" Davis)

One bookkeeper (known as "Ms. Mac")

. . . for a total of six employees. When Nancy looks back, she calls her tenure with the Drs. Stern "an opportunity of a lifetime. I learned from that experience that I could learn anything. It got my confidence up and my whole life's success goes back to Dr. Neuton Stern," she shares.

If Neuton began building his practice in 1920 on the pillars of uncommon patient care, research and technology, the 1950s reinforced that foundation when Tom Stern began practicing alongside his father. It was a solid foundation ripe to build on.

The Authors Stern

In the 1950s, Neuton and Tom Stern collaborated on more than professional practice; they authored a book together. It's telling that the book focuses on internal medicine rather than cardiology. Though some practice histories suggest that father and son phased out the internal medicine aspect of their practice in their first few years together, David Stern asserts: "My father insisted that he was an internist—not just a cardiologist. He was the equivalent of a primary care doctor for all of his patients."

Following is a list of books authored by Neuton and Tom Stern. Though all are out of print, and two remain unpublished, David keeps a robust collection on his bookshelf, and notices the tomes from time to time in other doctors' offices—particularly the text on physical diagnosis.

Clinical Diagnosis (1933)

Author: Neuton S. Stern, Publisher: Macmillan

The Bases of Treatment (1957)

Authors: Stern and Stern, Publisher: Charles C. Thomas

Clinical Examination: A Textbook of Physical Diagnosis (1964)

Author: Thomas N. Stern, Publisher: Year Book Medical Publishers

Rare Diseases in Internal Medicine (1966)

Author: Neuton S. Stern, Publisher: Charles C. Thomas

Understanding Sexual Behavior (1968), a pamphlet

Author: Neuton S. Stern

It is poignant to note that Neuton dedicated Rare Diseases in Internal Medicine to Tom with the following words: "To my son and confrere, Thomas N. Stern, upon whom I depend more than he realizes."

Similarly, Tom signed a copy of Clinical Examination given to his son with the words: "To my son David—with the hope that he will be as fine a physician as his grandfather." The message was dated August 28, 1985, on the occasion of David's first day of medical school at Vanderbilt University. David did go on to practice general internal medicine like his father and grandfather before him, though he also earned a doctoral degree in education from Stanford University. "My mother, father and grandfather were big educators, and I realized that I loved teaching too," explains David, who describes himself as "an educator and general internist." He currently serves as Chief of Medicine at the New York Harbor VA in Manhattan, home to 40,000 patients and 100 doctors; as Vice Chair for Education and Faculty Affairs at New York University; and as Co-Director of the Masters of Health Professions Education Program, a partnership between the NYU School of Medicine and Maastricht University in the Netherlands.

But back to the books: Neuton also wrote two unpublished works, one on philosophy and one on art (Art Appreciation and Criticism), evidence of his well-rounded interests. It's a trait he passed down to Tom, who once told colleague Randy Meeks that it was one of his biggest regrets not receiving a liberal arts education. Tom explained that his college years coincided with wartime and administrators were rushing students through the institution—he was only enrolled 18 months. Still, Randy remembers Tom Stern's "quick wit. He was one of the smartest people I've ever been around, but he was a renaissance man," she explains.

Photography was Tom Stern's true passion—one he shared with his daughter Carol—and he eventually took lessons from a friend, Murray Riss. Today, some of Tom's original photography decorates the patient floor of Stern Cardiovascular Foundation's main building.

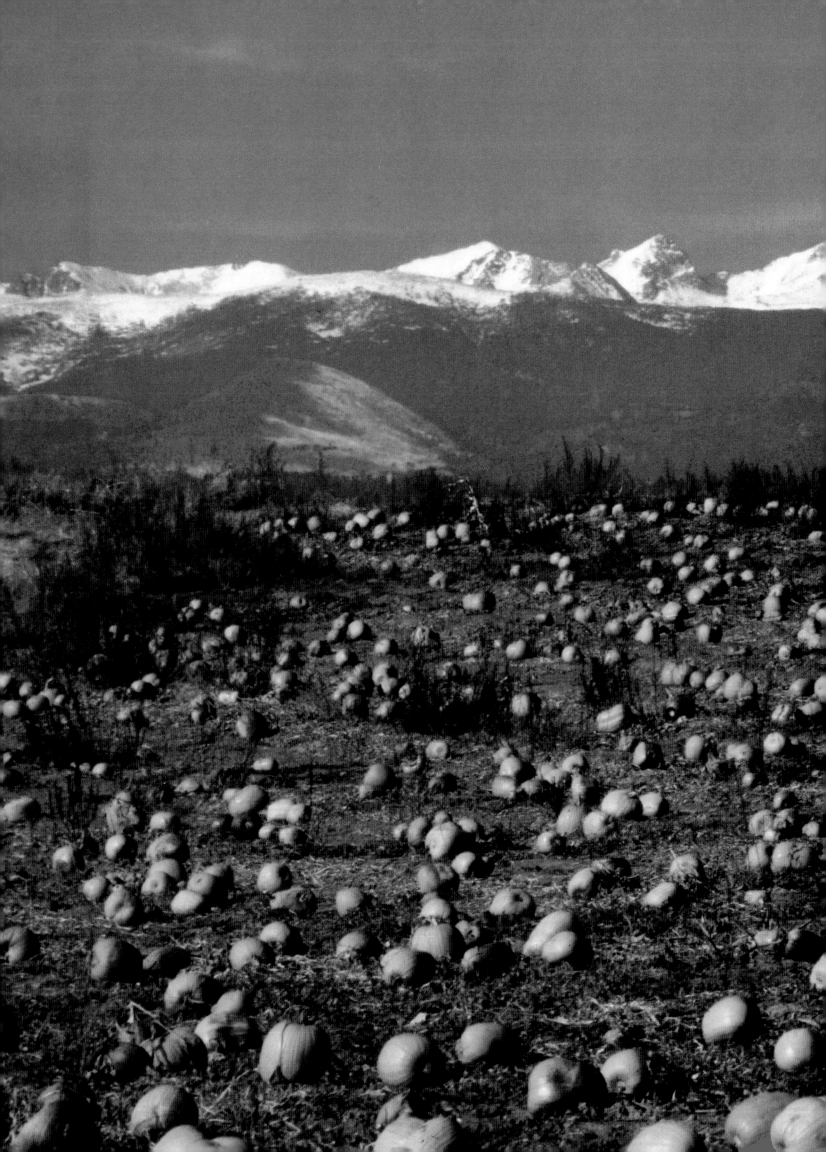

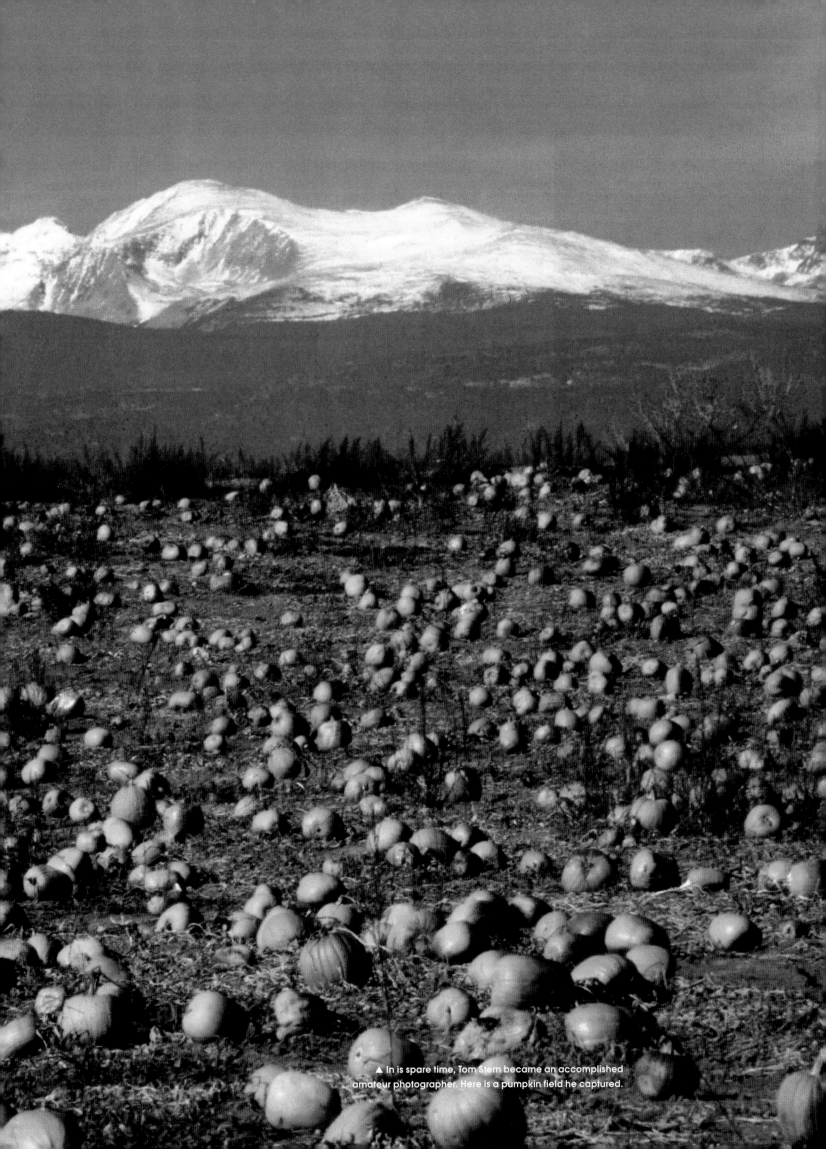

▲ In is spare time, Tom Stern became an accomplished amateur photographer. Here is a pumpkin field he captured.

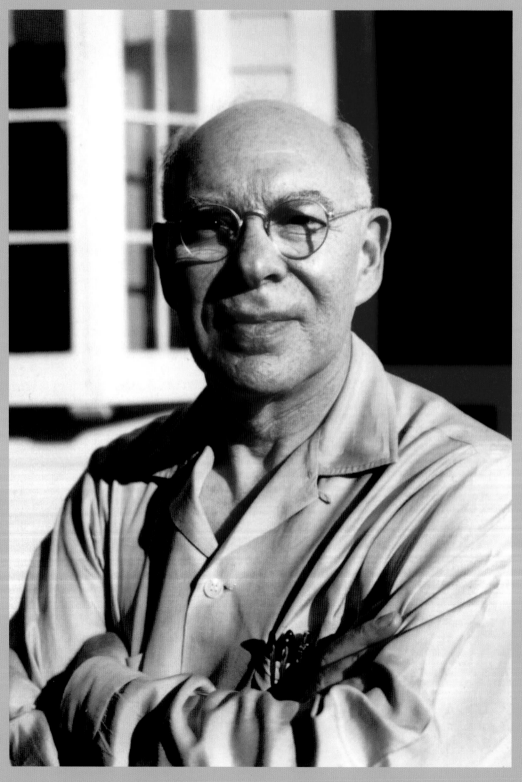

▲ Neuton Stern in the 1960s.

Photo courtesy of David Stern.

IN THE 1960S, A THIRD GENERATION OF STERNS BEGAN SPENDING TIME IN THE OFFICE: TOM'S CHILDREN AND THEIR COUSINS. SUSAN EDELMAN AND DAVID STERN ARE QUICK TO SHARE MEMORIES. AS DAVID TELLS IT, "MY DAD WOULD ALWAYS WORK ON SATURDAY MORNINGS—HE WOULD GO IN AND ROUND ON HIS PATIENTS. THE OFFICE WAS COMPLETELY EMPTY AND THE SIX OF US WOULD RUN AROUND PLAYING DOCTORS, PRETENDING WE WERE PATIENTS, WHILE WE WAITED FOR MY DAD TO FINISH HIS ROUNDS. THE REAL FUN WAS THE TREADMILL."

Weekdays, the atmosphere was more buttoned up.

Just after the turn of the new decade, the Sterns had recruited Nathan Salky into their practice. As Tom Stern recollected, "We had watched Nathan through residency, knowing him to be a brilliant young man and a very personable one. He came into the office after Army service." As their practice's capacity grew, so did their armamentarium:

In 1958, Frank Mason Sones Jr., M.D., of the Cleveland Clinic had inadvertently pioneered selective coronary angiography. Throughout the 1960s, the procedure came into increasing use; Tom reports that in the latter half of the decade, "left heart catheterizations were being done widely."

In 1964, H. Edward Garrett Sr., M.D., performed the world's first successful coronary artery bypass graft while working with Michael E. DeBakey, M.D., in Houston. (Garrett moved to Memphis a few years later to serve as Chairman of the Section of Cardiothoracic Surgery at the University of Tennessee.)

Furosemide was approved as a diuretic by the FDA in 1966, superseding harsh, unpredictable mercurials.

And, toward the end of the 1960s, "We were finally able to persuade Baptist to start its own laboratory," Tom reported, explaining:

"Dr. J. Leo Wright was brought down from Mayo Clinic to lead this. He was an excellent cardiologist and skillful at right heart catheterizations but was afraid to undertake left heart catheterization, then coming into common use. Baptist did not have left heart catheterizations until after his untimely death, and Frank Kroetz was brought in from the University of Iowa."

Kroetz would go on to serve as Director of Cardiac Laboratories at Baptist until 1990.

Indisputably, the 1960s were a time of great progress within the field of cardiology—the very origins of our acknowledgment of vascular surgery as a specialty in and of itself, supported by strides in diagnostics and therapies. In *Memphis Medicine: A History of Science and Service*, authors Patricia LaPointe McFarland and Mary Ellen Pitts consider how the progress hit home, summing up the era as follows: "[Eventually] imaging became part of treatment as well as diagnosis. Breakthrough diagnostic procedures changed cardiovascular medicine. Angiography improved the success of vascular surgical procedures of all types. Pioneers included Dr. Thomas Stern at Baptist."

Yet for all of its highs, the decade ended on a low. In July of 1969, Neuton Stern suffered his fatal heart attack. According to Tom, "Nathan Salky had just gone off for a two-week tour of Russia and Scandinavia. David Holloway had just joined us. Instead of coming to help out in a busy three-man office, [David] was suddenly left with the entire responsibility. He carried off his responsibility in a wonderful manner."

The Passing of a Patriarch

Neuton Stern's eulogy was delivered by the venerated Memphis Rabbi James A. Wax on July 15, 1969. On that day, Rabbi Wax said of Neuton:

"He had a prophetic concern for the welfare of others. He was sensitive to humanitarian needs; alert to social and moral responsibilities. His sympathies were with the unfortunate and the deprived. He was, indeed, a man of sterling character. He was a distinguished member of a distinguished calling. He had an exalted place in the medical profession. He was a scholar in the field of medicine.

And even as he brought healing to others, he found time to teach and to contribute to medical knowledge."

As previously mentioned, David Holloway joined the practice the very month that Neuton Stern passed away. He recollects that he logged about a week before Nathan Salky left for vacation and Neuton Stern went into the hospital, adding, "I was the lone sucker here. I didn't even know where the bathroom was, but I managed to work and see patients for about two weeks. That's quite a way to break in."

For Holloway, those two weeks in July of 1969 weren't just a crash course in practicing cardiology, they were a crash course in beginning to understand the legacy of Neuton Stern. "I knew Neuton Stern, but I didn't get to practice with him. I saw one of his patients and I had to inform this fellow—a working man—that Neuton had died. He broke down in tears. That's all I needed to know about Neuton," Holloway recalled.

Nathan Salky, M.D.

Tom Stern's description of Nathan Salky as "brilliant" was an apt one. Nathan ranked in the top of his medical school class and was a member of Alpha Omega Alpha Honor Medical Society (later,

▶ Drs. William L. Russo and David H. Holloway, Jr.

Photo credit: Stern Cardiovascular Foundation

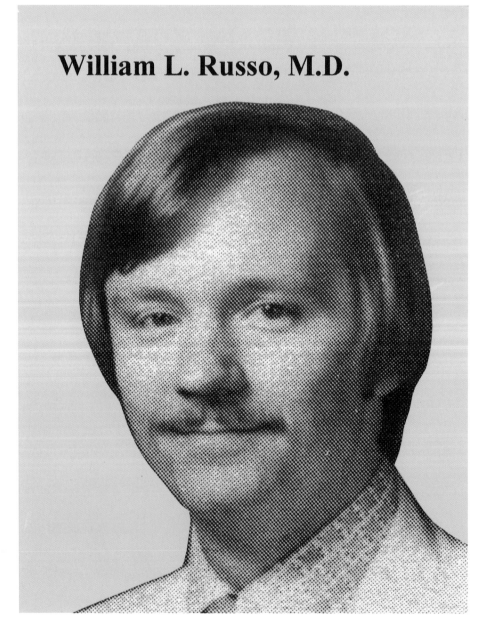

William L. Russo, M.D.

he became one of the first cardiologists in the Memphis area to become board-certified in cardiology).

Though Nathan was recruited to practice with Neuton and Tom in 1961 as a general cardiologist, he shared the Sterns' interest in research, and helped develop that capacity for the growing group. One of his most high-profile protocols was a double-blind study of an antiplatelet drug's effect on reinfarction. Sharon Goldstein, who was hired to the practice as Nathan's assistant on the study, remembers:

"He taught me everything I know. I was taught how to draw blood and take EKG readings. I had a portable EKG I would roll into the hospital and offer every person between the ages of 40 and 80 who had had a heart attack a free EKG. I would bring the charts back to Dr. Salky and he would determine who qualified to be on the study based on age, cardiac enzymes and so on. It was a godsend for the patients who qualified, as it meant they came every week to be seen by Dr. Salky. We watched them so carefully and they could call us at the drop of a hat. It was a national study and we got more patients enrolled than any other center in the country. From the study, Dr. Salky had papers published and went on a speaking tour."

To talk to those who worked alongside Nathan is to imagine a physician with an endearing, and enduring, bedside manner. As Brent Addington, M.D., reminisces: "He had a baritone voice so everyone seemed to listen to him, especially my 80-something-year-old grandmother. She would say, 'He is such a fine-looking gentleman.' The ladies also called him the 'Silver Fox.'" But, as Brent and others report, Nathan embodied style and substance: "He could get more patients to quit smoking than I had ever seen before using different techniques that always seemed to work," Brent notes.

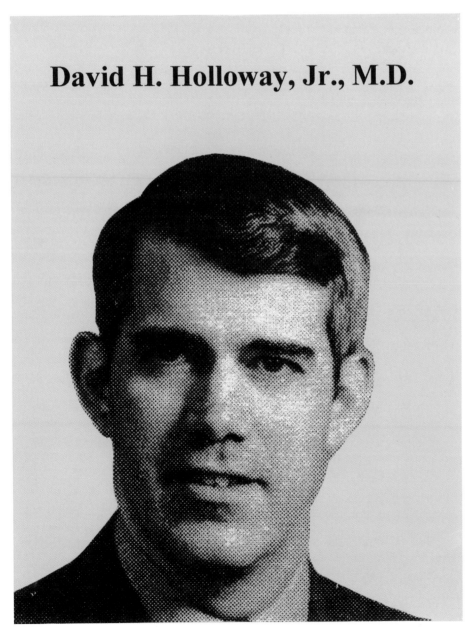

David H. Holloway, Jr., M.D.

Randy Meeks, who served as Nathan's nurse until he left the practice, may sum his legacy up best: "Dr. Salky was not only a very popular doctor with employees, hospital staff and patients, he was a well-known and beloved Memphian," she offers.

After 20-plus years with the practice, Nathan Salky left to wind down—while helping to build up the next generation of cardiologists in Memphis. In 1985, he began consulting for two young cardiologists in town, Drs. Brent Addington and Ray Allen, Jr. The two have since joined the Stern fold.

Nathan Salky—cardiologist, researcher, mentor and aficionado of tennis and sailing—passed away in 1990, survived by his wife and two adult children.

Sincere thanks to Brent Addington, M.D., Cynthia Bicknell, Randy Meeks and Sharon Goldstein for contributing to this profile.

David Holloway, M.D.

"David Holloway is the Tom Brady of Stern Cardiovascular Foundation." —Steven Gubin, M.D., President, Stern Cardiovascular Foundation

Like Neuton and Tom before him, David Holloway arrived at professional practice by way of the United States Armed Forces. The Tennessee native completed his undergraduate studies at the University of Chattanooga before advancing to medical school at the University of Tennessee and medical training at Duke University Medical Center. Then duty called. At the School of Aerospace Medicine in San Antonio, the

newly trained cardiologist evaluated pilots for health problems. "I came right out of the Air Force to practice . . . I've never taken time off to find myself," Holloway likes to say.

Tom Stern happened to be teaching a few courses during David's enrollment at the University of Tennessee. "I knew his father was a revered cardiologist in town," Holloway remembers. But Holloway had North Carolina on his mind, feeling a loyalty to the area where he had completed his fellowship and residency. As he remembers, the area around Duke:

". . . was a much more appealing area than Memphis at the time, but I did come over and talk to Tom and Nathan. It was right after Dr. Martin Luther King Jr.'s assassination. [Tom's] father was with us; he was a grand fellow. I had actually joined a practice in Raleigh but it kept nagging me that this was the right place, so I called Tom and wound up here. I knew him as a professor at the University [of Tennessee]. I wanted to come back for him, not for the city."

At the onset, David made some astounding diagnoses, including one involving a patient of Tom Stern's. When David told the patient to report to the hospital, she responded in a way he has never forgotten: "She said, 'Now go check with Dr. Tom because you're wet behind the ears and I don't trust you.' She was my patient for the rest of her life. But everybody loved Tom. He was a compassionate doctor. He always took patients into his office and talked with them about things outside of the exam room. He was an inspiration in the way he practiced," David asserts.

David Holloway would go on to serve as president of the group—third in succession following Neuton and Tom Stern, from 1992 to 2008—and, for Baptist Memorial Hospital, as Secretary, Chief and President of Staff, as well as a member of the Board of Trustees and several committees (through the early- to mid-1980s). Now in his fifth decade at the practice, David has the perspective to consider how things have changed, both within the field and within the microcosm of Stern. As he shares, "It's totally different from what I learned training at Duke. We do caths and open those up immediately to prevent heart attack, rather than keep patients in bed. We have electrical means of controlling the heart. If the heart's fast, with a fibrillator, we can go in and freeze it. It's progressed remarkably and it's easy except for computer work," David laughs.

As for how things have changed within the ecosystem of the practice, David explains that by the current organizational structure, there are three to four doctors in a pod, plus secretaries, nurses and a pacer. "We're as close in our own group as I was back then, when there were only five of us in the office, and my patients are still friends. That's a good relationship," muses the 82-year-old, who still sees patients daily. "You just start working and you keep working . . . that's the secret," he shares.

Full Circle

Fifty years after Tom Stern's patient called David Holloway "wet behind the ears," Jennifer Morrow, M.D., notices a similar reaction by the patients of David

Holloway and his peers to the practice's younger generation of doctors. "The older guys don't go to the hospital anymore, so the younger doctors go for them. Their patients will say, 'Can you just run this by Dr. Holloway?'" she laughs. When the new generation obliges, they get a glimpse of David's knowledge and recall of patients, Morrow explains. "You'll say, 'I promised your patient I would touch base with you,' and he knows everything about that patient without opening a chart or a computer," she says.

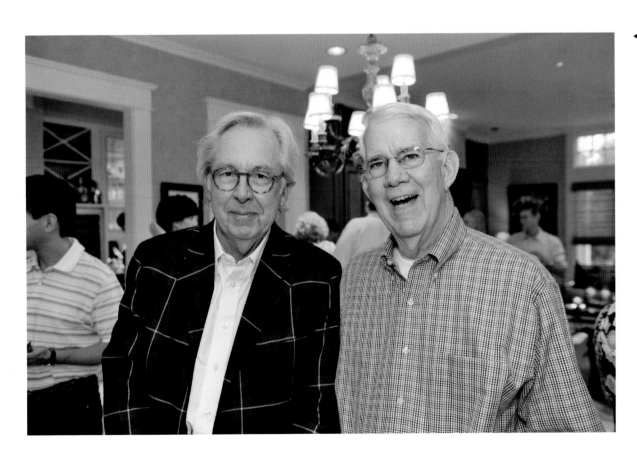

◀ Left to right: Dr. Frank McGrew and Dr. David H. Holloway, Jr.

Photo credit: Stern Cardiovascular Foundation

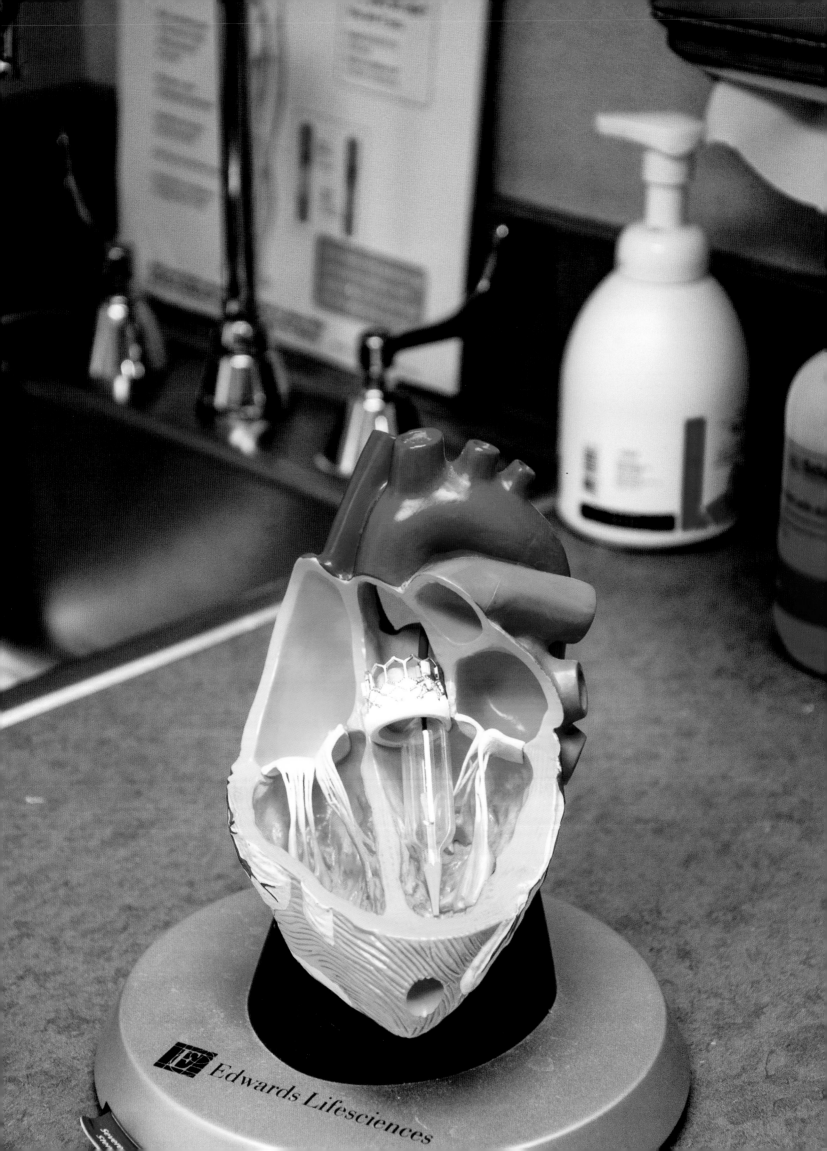

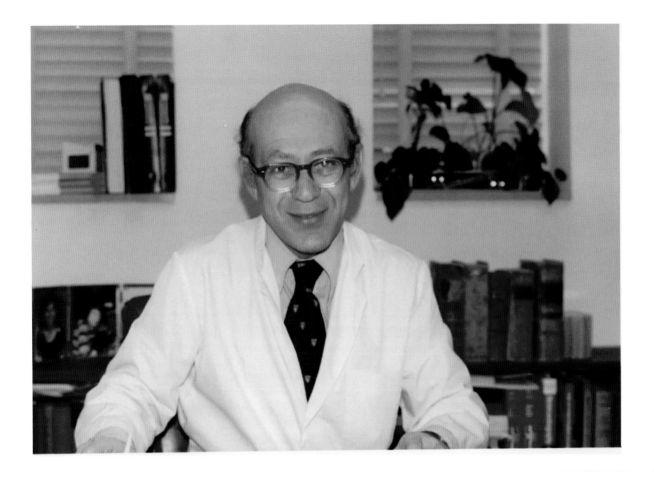

▲ Tom Stern
Photo thanks to Randy Meeks

L IKE THE 1960S, THE 1970S WERE A TIME OF PROGRESS FOR BOTH THE PRACTICE OF CARDIOLOGY AND THE PRACTICE OF TOM STERN.

The practice Tom's father founded 50 years earlier as a one-man endeavor would emerge from the decade six doctors and five employees strong. "We stayed very busy. When I started practice, we had perhaps 10 patients in the hospital between the two of us," Tom Stern recounted in his retrospective, recalling the days of practicing alongside his father. "By the 1970s," he continued, "the doctor on call for the weekend would have 100 to 140 patients on the hospital list."

In response, the practice began recruiting. Frank McGrew and William Russo joined in 1976; Jan Turner in 1978 (see individual biographies at the end of this chapter). "We built on a very firm foundation," David Holloway explains of the practice's recruitment efforts.

From new employees including Sharon Goldstein to summer helpers like Susan Edelman, answering the phone at this time became arduous. "We answered the phone 'Stern, Salky, Holloway, Russo and McGrew' back then," Sharon remembers.

"Then we added 'Turner' to the end of it and the people answering the phones said 'We can't do this anymore.' We decided we were going to have to simplify our name," Jan Turner remembers.

And that's how, in the final year of the decade, Stern, Salky, Holloway, Russo, McGrew and Turner became the Cardiology Group of Memphis (CGoM).

Building a Support Staff

Accordingly, the group grew its office staff. In 1974, Randy Meeks answered an ad in the newspaper with the following description: "Girl Friday, venipuncture, EKG, X-ray; will train." At the time, Randy was attending college without a clear picture of what she wanted to do with her schooling. What she certainly couldn't have envisioned was that, out of 100 applicants who would send letters to Drs. Stern, Salky and Holloway in response to that newspaper ad, she would be the one chosen. Nor could she have foreseen what that decision would mean for her professional and personal growth. To start, she'd work as a medical assistant in the lab. Even then, she says, with less than 15 people in the entire office, "It was busy. It's always been busy."

Nancy Cummings started in July 1976, the same month that Drs. Russo and McGrew joined. As the group's only full-time medical transcriptionist, Nancy admits to feeling, "somewhat overwhelmed . . . there was so much work," even with the ultramodern automatic typewriter she was given to complete her job. Still, Nancy persisted, becoming supervisor over all of the group's medical transcription—and Tom Stern's personal transcriptionist. "His initial evaluations would sometimes be three pages long. I would go over the letters after I would type them but occasionally [an error] would slip through and he would always make a mark," she recalls, chuckling. Between transcriptions, Nancy would often round with doctors at the hospital. She wasn't a nurse, though she dreamed of becoming one.

Sharon Goldstein was hired in 1976 as well. Despite her degrees in English and theatre (from Vanderbilt University), she soon began functioning as Jan Turner's assistant—not unlike Nancy Cummings. "I was taking blood and blood pressure, doing EKGs, going to the hospital to make rounds . . . I functioned that way for a long time," Sharon reminisces. When her role in the practice transitioned, she laughs, "I had a lot of physicians from other offices saying, 'Did they fire you as a nurse? I would like to hire you!'"

Echoing Sharon, Randy remembers, "There were no nurses at the practice then. We drew the blood, shot chest X-rays, did minor blood tests, ran EKGs, put people in rooms and worked them up for the doctors like a medical assistant does now."

Two of the practice's original "para-nurses," Randy Meeks and Nancy Cummings, would learn they had a knack for the vocation. Randy would complete her schooling in the 1980s; Nancy in the 1990s.

Randy remembers the moment her new path came into focus. "I heard the doctors whispering to each other about hiring some nurses and I decided: If they were going to hire nurses, that is what I wanted to do. Dr. Stern knew that I had applied and been accepted to nursing school and he had been on the phone with someone about a Holter monitor—we had a couple of monitors and would take the tapes to the hospital to be read; he was talking to someone about acquiring a machine to read our own. And I said, 'Are we getting a Holter machine?' And he said, 'I have to find something for you to

do while you go back to nursing school,'" she remembers with a smile in her voice.

Tom adhered to his plan. Once Randy began her formal training, she says: "I couldn't be there every day from nine to five like I was usually, so during breaks between semesters I would be there every day. The office was open Saturdays, 9 a.m. - 1 p.m., for people who had to work. The staff rotated to cover those days and I worked every one. Having the Holter machine meant I could do the tapes anytime. I would also come in any night when school was done and make scan tapes for hours."

A "Panoply of Tools"

In addition to increasing its bandwidth, the practice increased its adoption of what Tom Stern referred to as "the panoply of tools of the electrophysiologist." He elaborated on the contents of this toolbox in his retrospective:

"Other oral medications appeared on the scene with varying success as we learned more and more about their good and bad effects. The first major therapeutic advance was in the use of beta blockers started in the 1970s."

"The 1970s were an exciting time in cardiology," Jan Turner echoes. In addition to a number of new, effective medicines—he cites ACE inhibitors in addition to beta blockers—Baptist Memorial Hospital was a magnet for talent. "We had Ed Garrett Sr., Ed Garrett Jr. and Rodney Wolf, so we had first-class surgeons," Jan recalls. The result: "The incidence of death from cardiovascular disease significantly diminished. That was a fun time to be in our field in

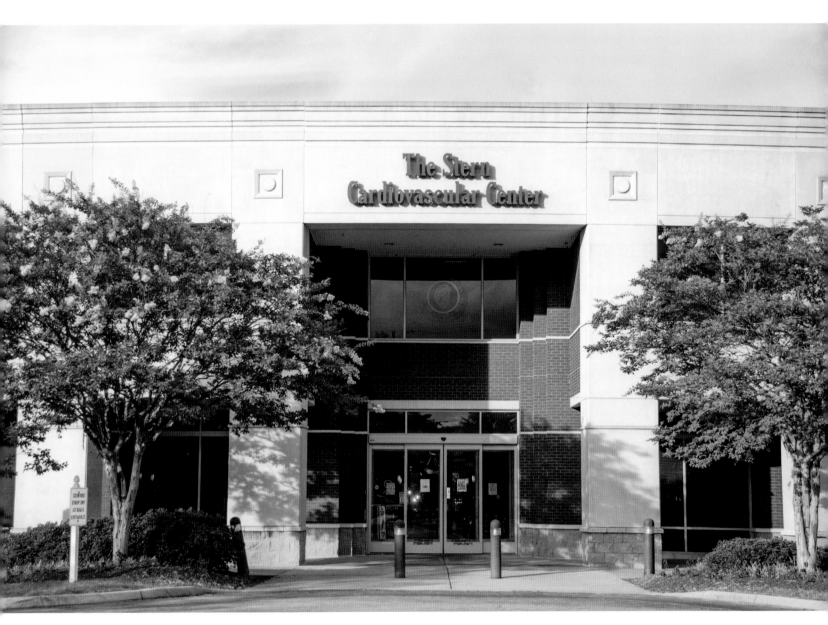

▲ The Stern Cardiovascular Foundation

Photo by Stephanie Norwood

Memphis and across the country," Jan asserts.

On the state of imaging in the 1970s, Tom noted:

"We moved to radionuclide stress testing and echocardiographic stress testing. The most recent technologic step, of course, was the CT scanner."

As you'll learn in Jan Turner's biography at the end of this chapter, cardiac ultrasound imaging was one of the tools he added to the panoply when he joined the group in 1978.

In *Memphis Medicine: A History of Science and Service*, authors McFarland and Pitts summarize that the 1970s marked the period when "Memphis medicine became increasingly sub-specialized." David Holloway remembers it well. When he joined the practice in 1969, "we were the only cardiologists around. Within eight or nine years, that changed," he explains. The trend, no coincidence, ran concurrent with the "era of more precise diagnostic medicine, led by developments in imaging," (McFarland & Pitts, 2011). The authors go on to name Thomas Stern as leading the local vanguard.

It is telling that in a 1993 profile of Tom Stern published in The Commercial Appeal, writer Mary Powers defines the term "cardiologist" for readers.

What's more, Tom and his colleagues were providing more to their patients than mere diagnosis and medical management. As Tom noted, "Defibrillation became routine when needed in the early 1970s and right-sided pacemakers—first temporary, then permanent—were implanted." The

decade also saw the acceptance of coronary artery bypass graft surgery as treatment and the advent of catheter-based interventions, including an idea advanced by one Andreas Gruentzig, M.D. Before a skeptical group of physicians at a meeting of the American Heart Association in 1975, Gruentzig shared the idea of using balloon catheters to dilate coronary arteries. The episode calls to mind Neuton Stern's presentation of the electrocardiogram some 50 years prior. Yet, supporting physicians rallied around Gruentzig and the first balloon angioplasty procedure on a coronary artery was performed in 1977, marking a breakthrough in interventional cardiology.

One angle that gets overlooked when we focus on technological advances is the nature of what it was like to practice in the era under examination. Aided by hindsight, Frank McGrew compares the 1970s to the present day: "It was easy initially. We just had the one big hospital with 2,000 beds—the largest private hospital in the world—everything under one roof. There wasn't a lot of competition between groups. But on the other hand, it was a lot harder. We didn't have nurse practitioners, well-trained emergency room doctors, hospital assistants or cell phones."

PRACTICING TECHNOLOGY

While the Cardiology Group of Memphis was able to fully conduct several diagnostic procedures—from performing the tests to interpreting test results—this was not the norm for practices in the 1970s. As such, CGoM

physicians were regularly enlisted to read EKGs performed in other facilities. Susan Edelman remembers working at the practice over summer breaks from high school at the time:

"I was at the bottom of the totem pole, but in summer, everybody would move up a notch. I would file and answer the EKG. Hospitals that were in north Mississippi, eastern Arkansas or even counties around Shelby County had no one who could read EKGs. But there was a way to transmit the EKG over a phone line. When those locations were going to do an EKG, they would call and identify themselves. We would plug the phone into a device that would print out the EKG in the Stern office. This was pre-fax, pre-computer, but those results would be transmitted from these outlying hospitals to our office; a Stern doctor would read them and send a report to the hospital."

Other CGoM employees remember a computer nicknamed George, the first office computer for which Tom advocated. David Stern doesn't remember the name George, but, he notes, "I absolutely remember punch cards. My father would come home with this stack of punch cards the size of a folded-up envelope. Around the edges of the cards were holes and if you punched through the outer rim, the hole became a notch. Different areas around the [perimeter] of the card were associated with different things they wanted to keep track of for patients." Susan didn't remember George by name either, but she was sure of one thing: "My father was interested in anything new, and any good technology that helped anybody was important to him."

Back to School

David Stern has another strong memory of his father's professional life in the 1970s: Tom Stern studying to be recertified by the American Board of Internal Medicine (ABIM):

"There was a time you took a board certification in medicine and you were considered to be board-certified for the rest of your life. We call it the ballistic model of education: We give you a lot of education early on. In about 1978, they started thinking about retesting people who had already certified. They put out a request for people to participate in a pilot. The results would be inconsequential, but they wanted to see how physicians would perform. My father insisted on taking it. I was studying for Advanced Placement Biology or Chemistry in high school, and I remember my father studying for his boards because he wanted to be certified in internal medicine, not just cardiology."

Susan Edelman, too, remembers her father studying, and adds another dimension to his motivation. "He felt very strongly that all physicians should be board-certified, and he wasn't going to ask people to do something that he was not going to do," she explains.

Lessons from Tom Stern

After Nancy Cummings began working as a nurse for CGoM, she encountered a patient with supraventricular tachycardia (SVT) during night call. She remembered something Tom Stern had told her in the office one day. "Go and get a large pan and fill it with ice and put some water in it. Let it get cold. Put the patient's face in the ice water. You have to crawl down in there like a polar bear," she recalls Tom instructing. She shared Tom's tip with her patient's family and checked back after a half-hour. "That broke it," she reports.

Direct, no-nonsense advice: If this was one of Tom Stern's trademarks, it was undoubtedly inspired by his father. (Maybe you recall the story from the 1950s of Neuton Stern advising any patient who wouldn't change his or her lifestyle to find another doctor.) Regardless, Susan Edelman saw it play out at her father's office and at home. As she explains: "We had two rules growing up: You could not smoke tobacco and you could not ride a motorcycle. People had just started to understand tobacco as a cause of heart attack as my father was beginning to practice. If he wanted you to quit smoking and you'd say, 'I'll try,' he'd say, 'NO. Just do it.' He was very self-assured and could be stern. But he meant for things to be done properly."

Frank McGrew, M.D.

"In the field of heart failure, there are several medications and devices that are part of standardized care. Every major type of pacemaker or defibrillator, every drug that's been approved for heart failure—at least 20 if not more of the drugs and devices—we've done clinical trials in every one. What that means is, if you came to the Research Department at Stern, you received advanced care often several years before those solutions were available to the general community." —Frank McGrew, M.D.

Amid the clinical notes of Tom Stern's retrospective lies this gem on staffing: "Frank McGrew was told by people at Duke about this crazy practice in Memphis, so he came to see us." Tom's original plan had been to hire just one additional physician, and William Russo had already been recruited to fill the spot. Nevertheless, Tom noted, "We decided Frank was too good to pass up." Here's the story of how that came to pass.

Before completing his residency and fellowship at Duke University Medical Center, Frank McGrew received his undergraduate degree from Johns Hopkins University and his medical degree from Case Western Reserve University. "When I finished training, the extra year training in different disciplines wasn't done," Frank explains. Yet, he was drawn to conduct research on rhythm abnormalities and heart failure. That led to a fellowship in the Heart Rhythm Society, the Heart Failure Society of America, the American Heart Association and the American College of Cardiology. "It was uncommon to have fellowships in all four of these groups," Frank asserts, and yet, "In one year or another, I had presented papers at the national meetings of all of these organizations. There was also a European rhythm society, the European Heart Rhythm Association. I lectured there twice in addition to doing posters and things as a member of the society," he reports.

Frank describes himself as someone who's at home in a research environment. At the age of 16, he entered a Westinghouse Science Talent Search (now the Regeneron Science Talent Search), assisted by Melvin Calvin. "I won the science fair and he won the Nobel Prize," Frank laughs, referring to Calvin's 1961 capture of the Nobel Prize in Chemistry. Frank also gained experience working with Joseph Goldstein, M.D., at the National Heart Institute in Bethesda, Maryland. (Goldstein would win the Nobel Prize in Physiology or Medicine in 1985, with Michael S. Brown, "for their discoveries concerning the regulation of cholesterol metabolism," creating the model for the modern-day treatment of hyperlipidemia.) Frank's family history sparked his curiosity as well: After his father was diagnosed with heart disease, Frank may have asked a question or two of the family doctor.

Remember Paul Dudley White, classmate and Army buddy of Neuton Stern? "When I was at Duke," Frank explains, "it was the world center for Wolff-Parkinson-White (WPW) syndrome [a condition characterized by abnormal electrical pathways in the heart]. Three people were given credit for discovering the condition. One was Paul Dudley White. Talk about being in the right place at the right time," Frank muses.

Frank's interest in research and active, prolific scholarship enabled him to fit right into the culture of a medical practice cultivated by Neuton and Tom Stern. As Frank explains: "When I came [to Memphis], I saw that Thomas Stern had patients in the hospital who were relatives of the faculty members at the university. He encouraged research." And though Frank didn't have the chance to work alongside Neuton Stern, he was aware that Neuton and Tom had studied digitalis together.

At the same time, Frank saw that Nathan Salky was actively engaged in heart attack research. "The fact that Nathan was doing that

convinced me that this place was fertile for doing research," Frank remembers.

Witnessing the work of Tom and Nathan, Frank determined, "Anywhere that had that much emphasis on research was a place I wanted to be." Frank acknowledges that factors outside of the practice helped decide him, as well:

"When I was looking at jobs around the country, Baptist Memorial Hospital was the largest private hospital. There was some research going on then—really limited, but it was a start. I saw that this would be a great place to practice and research without some of the encumberments that come with a full-fledged academic practice. If I stayed at Duke, by convention I would have focused on research in one area; that's the nature of the academic institution. But here, I could research a broad spectrum."

That, he did. Of his early days at the practice, Frank remembers, "I was encouraged to do anything I wanted in terms of research. When I first came and there were just five physicians, I could count on all five of us—any patient that showed up would be an appropriate person to put in a research project."

Over time, Frank followed his passion into the role of Director of Clinical Research for Stern Cardiovascular. He drew on previous experience coordinating multi-center research studies for the National Heart Institute to deepen Stern's commitment to research. While Frank doesn't count the number of studies or patients touched by Stern's research initiatives, he's voluble when it comes to discussing highlights of

his oeuvre. It's poignant to note the scope of these highlights, considering Frank's initial decision to join Stern for its wide-open approach to research. "Through the years, I've been able to do research in every area of cardiology," he affirms, from implanting the first two-lead pacemaker in the city of Memphis to undertaking a recent study of a four-lead pacemaker, and conducting trials of almost every new drug to advance the field in the last 40 years.

"When I first came [to Stern], patients with heart failure were so sick. They couldn't breathe; they couldn't walk far; they were exhausted all the time. They had to take a lot of medication. Now, you can't pick them out of a crowd. Thanks to Dr. McGrew's research, step by step, we've opened doors for patients, offering treatment they would not have gotten had they not been at Stern. Heart disease has come such a long way and Dr. Mcgrew had a huge impact." —Elissa Fine, Lipid Clinic Coordinator, Stern Cardiovascular Foundation

It requires a concerted effort within Stern to bring research study opportunities to patients. Frank currently oversees two research teams—one at Stern's main office and one on-site at Baptist—involving, among others, physicians, research nurses and admins, a nurse practitioner and a physician assistant. "It takes a village. We couldn't function without the entire team considering the regulatory documents, lab work and scheduling," Frank explains. Adding to the daily workload, Frank's team stays active sharing its research findings. "We've had several talks and publications going back 20-some years.

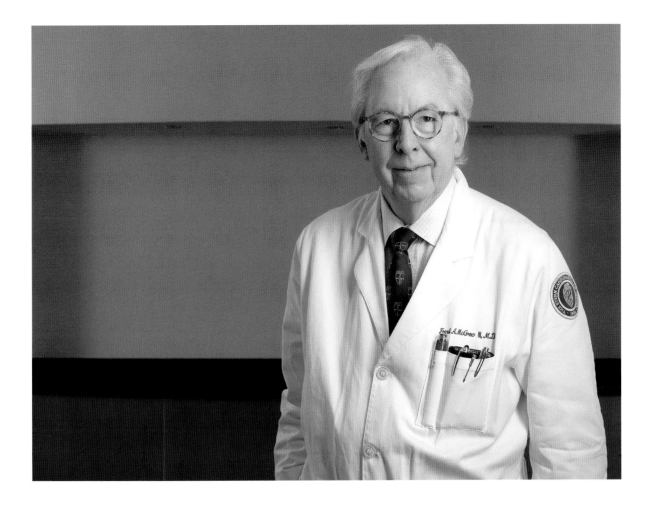

◀ Dr. Frank McGrew

Photo credit: Stern Cardio

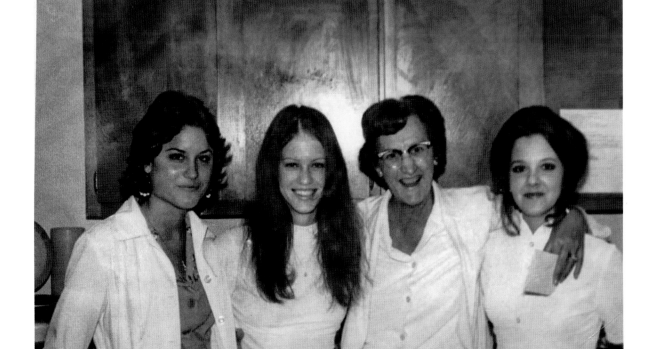

◀ Diane Moody, Randy
Meeks, Mildred Chambers,
and Beth Reynolds in 1974.

Photo thanks to Randy Meeks.

1974

There are four major meetings in the U.S.: the Heart Rhythm Society, the Heart Failure Society of America, the American College of Cardiology and the American Heart Association. We've had presentations at all of those. We've also made a presentation to the European Society of Cardiology, the largest cardiology organization in the world," Frank says.

All the while, Frank has never wavered in his personal commitment to professional development, or to the development of others. He has held several academic appointments, including clinical assistant professor of medicine in the Division of Cardiology for Duke University Clinical Cardiology Studies and associate clinical professor at the University of Tennessee College of Health Sciences. Most recently, Frank was one of five Stern physicians to earn heart failure certification, a new sub-specialty. Incidentally, he happened to admit the first patient to Baptist Memorial Hospital East some 40 years ago. "I remember it well," Frank begins, continuing, "It was a fellow that had an overdose of a heart medication called quinidine, which is very rare."

The foundational research of Neuton and Tom Stern, built on by the work of Nathan Salky, Frank McGrew and a new generation of Stern support staff and physicians, including Drs. Eric Johnson and Mark Coppess, has contributed significantly to the advancement of cardiac treatment and the improvement of patient outcomes.

While this dedication to staying at the forefront of cardiovascular research is rooted in the history of the practice, Frank believes it will be just as fundamental to its future. "Cardiac treatments have improved dramatically, but there is residual risk," he explains. There is also hope, thanks to the Research Team of Stern Cardiovascular Foundation.

WILLIAM RUSSO, M.D.

William Russo was well known to Drs. Tom Stern, Nathan Salky and David Holloway following his outstanding academic achievements as a medical student, intern, resident and cardiology fellow at the University of Tennessee. William "Bill" Russo accepted a position to join the group in 1976.

Bill's practice rapidly expanded, in part because he became interested in the non-cardiac causes of chest pain and mitral valve prolapse. At the time, the two factors were common areas of cardiac referrals that were just beginning to be understood and characterized. Bill's efforts to treat and explain these conditions to patients were important, as good treatment protocols were unavailable.

As cardiac ultrasound (echocardiography) became increasingly more important in the noninvasive evaluation of patients during the 1970s, Bill stepped up again. As both the technical capabilities of the equipment and the expertise of the interpreters improved, cardiac structures could be quite accurately imaged. Crucial data concerning cardiac function could be obtained, which facilitated better treatment and evaluation. Bill would become an integral part of the practice's ultrasound department.

Throughout his career, Bill was recognized as one of the outstanding clinical cardiologists in the Mid-South. He showed a consistent, genuine dedication to the improvement of his patients' health, along with a similar focus on the quality of care rendered by the practice as a whole. To this end, Bill served in leadership positions throughout his career, and his input was crucial to the growth and development of the practice. He retired in July 2019.

"Bill Russo was the quintessential team player: looking after his patients and responsibilities; willing to help with any other tasks or colleagues' patients. If someone was sick or detained by an emergency in the hospital, you could count on his assistance," notes Jan Turner, M.D.

Sincere thanks to Jan Turner, M.D., for contributing this profile.

JAN TURNER, M.D.

Jan Turner was still associated with Emory University in 1977 when he first came to Memphis. He'll never forget his first day in the city: August 16, 1977, the day Elvis Presley died.

Jan was in town because a professor of his at Emory was a friend of Nathan Salky. Nathan extended an invitation for Jan to visit Memphis through their mutual acquaintance. What happened upon Jan's arrival was entirely unexpected:

"As luck would have it, we were rounding at Baptist. Nathan was showing me around and got an emergency call—they wanted him to come resuscitate Elvis. Nathan went down there and returned 45 minutes or so later and said Elvis had died. They did the autopsy—Eric Muirhead, head of pathology at UT and several of his colleagues—and Jerry Francisco, the county coroner, observed. To everyone's surprise, Francisco announced the death was due to cardiac arrhythmia. So that was my first day in Memphis."

Before the first anniversary of Elvis' death, Jan Turner would join Salky et al. in Memphis. Considering the drama of Jan's first visit to the city, what attracted him? As he explains:

"I had looked at several practices and thought about staying at Emory. But I liked the set-up. The practice was obviously growing, so that was a positive for me. Another important thing from my standpoint: I had done some early ultrasound work at the University of Colorado and some at Emory and was interested in continuing that. The group did not have a cardiac ultrasound lab and they were excited about me starting that.

"Baptist was also a plus. It was just Baptist Central back then, the largest private hospital in the country. They had state-of-the-art equipment in the operating rooms as well as in the cath labs. Ed Garrett was there, who had performed the first coronary bypass operation in Houston. At that time, the hospital was the primary teaching facility for the University of Tennessee, so we had med students, interns, fellows and residents all rotating through our services. I was anxious to continue with a teaching sort of institution."

Inside the practice, Jan recognized "another plus: They had long been involved in clinical cardiac research. Stern and Salky managed most of that, but as I came, Frank McGrew took that over. This initiative was subsidized by the

group because it kept them on the cutting-edge and allowed patients to benefit from the latest treatments," Jan explains.

Considering these factors holistically, Jan made his decision. "This was precisely the sort of thing I wanted. That's how I ended up in Memphis," he shares.

As anticipated, Jan began contributing his cardiac ultrasound capabilities to the group. "At that time, people were just beginning to use intravenous nitroglycerin. We had used that, along with other similar drugs, at Emory, so my new partners were anxious to get involved in that," Jan explains. Yet, he faced some opposition initially. "The pharmacy and nursing staff were afraid they would blow up if they dropped a bag, but the form of nitroglycerin used in medicine is modified relative to the type used in dynamite. It took a little time to convince everybody," Jan laughs.

Cardiac ultrasound wasn't the sole area Jan helped the group explore. At Emory, Jan had been involved in projects analyzing sudden death in young athletes. Hypertrophic cardiomyopathy was the leading cause of death among this population, and Jan began to give talks on the subject throughout the Mid-South and Midwest. "The main thrust was to educate primary care physicians on what to look for and ask about when they were doing teen physicals for sports teams," Jan explains.

One year after Jan joined the Cardiology Group of Memphis, Baptist Memorial Hospital East opened. CGoM opened a satellite location there, and Jan was tasked with running it. The post was another outward symbol of Jan's deep connection to the hospital.

Its presence had helped recruit him to Memphis, and now Baptist would serve as a proving ground for Jan's growing interest in scholarship and leadership.

"I always particularly enjoyed the teaching aspect of our practice and working with the students, residents and so forth. I found that I learned interesting tidbits from them—it forced you to keep up with the current medical literature," Jan shares. At the time, Baptist was Memphis' major clinical teaching hospital. "The University of Tennessee only had 300 or 400 beds. They didn't have the money or technology that Baptist had," Jan explains. Thus, Jan began teaching in the Baptist system as a clinical associate professor of medicine. He was awarded Most Outstanding Attending Physician for 1989-1990.

Around the same time, Jan served on the hospital board, becoming its Vice Chief of Staff in 1993. He remained equally engaged within CGoM, serving as the group's vice president to David Holloway. "It was a real honor to work with him and call him a colleague. David is just a first-rate guy," Jan reflects.

For all of the work, Jan remembers the laughs. As he shares:

"In the late 1970s or early 1980s, Tom, Bill Russo and myself were seeing patients together in Baptist Central, our main office at that time. A lady appeared at the check-in desk and told the person manning it that a man had passed out and fallen out of his chair in the waiting room. The clerk called for an emergency—docs stat to the waiting room—and the three physicians there headed up. Tom was closest to the door. By the time Bill and I got there, Tom had picked this patient up and carried him to McGrew's room where we could work on him. This shocked me because Tom was not a weight-lifter—he had a slight build. I couldn't believe he got this guy in McGrew's office before we could even get there. [The man] was not a patient of ours; he was the husband of a patient who was in with Tom Stern. We resuscitated the guy and it had a happy ending: We got him into the hospital and a couple weeks later, he walked out. But the other part that was interesting for Tom, Bill and I was that we had totally trashed McGrew's office. He was out of town and this was on a Friday. We had hundreds of feet of EKG tracings, IV tubing and oxygen tubing . . . Frank never had a tidy office; I always thought it was a fire hazard. So we decided to close Frank's door and put a sign on it not to clean his room. The next Monday, McGrew comes strolling in from his vacation, goes and sits down at his desk and doesn't even recognize it wasn't the same way he left it."

Some years later, Jan admits that he, along with Drs. Holloway and Gubin, were cited by the Health Care Financing Administration (HCFA) for unreadable handwriting. (Today, the federal organization is known as the Centers for Medicare and Medicaid Services.) The citations required remediation: The offending physicians would have to have their hospital notes typed for six months, during which time they would complete a compulsory course in handwriting. "The course we took was proctored by an elementary school teacher. We had to write sentences like, 'Jack and Jill ran up the hill, but Spot fell down' repeatedly," Jan relays.

For Jan, the punishment sparked clever problem-solving. "I came up with a patient encounter form that was mostly typed; you could check boxes," Jan explains, as opposed to entering longer-form notes by hand. HCFA was not amused, at least initially. The organization refused to accept Jan's form. In time, however, the practice received notification that a suspiciously similar-looking form was acceptable. It seems as though Jan's template made an impression.

Before Jan shared this story, the matter of his handwriting had already surfaced in the course of conducting interviews for this book. From Nancy Cummings:

"I remember the Christmas before Dr. Turner joined the group, we received a Christmas card from him with his children playing in the snow. We were all so excited about the new doctor, even though those of us in medical transcription were a little bewildered by his handwriting."

Author's note: I received a personal missive from Jan Turner enclosed with a Commercial Appeal article he wished to share on Tom Stern. Though Jan closed the note with the sentiment, "I hope you can read this!!" I found his handwriting to be perfectly legible.

Though Jan retired from Stern Cardiovascular Center in 2006, he keeps tabs on the practice and likes what he sees. "I look at the medical training and the academic achievements of the new folks. I counted the number of languages spoken by the physicians recently and it's 15. I'm still struggling to be proficient in my native language," he jests. In all seriousness, Jan adds, "I feel very fortunate to

have worked with such a dedicated group."

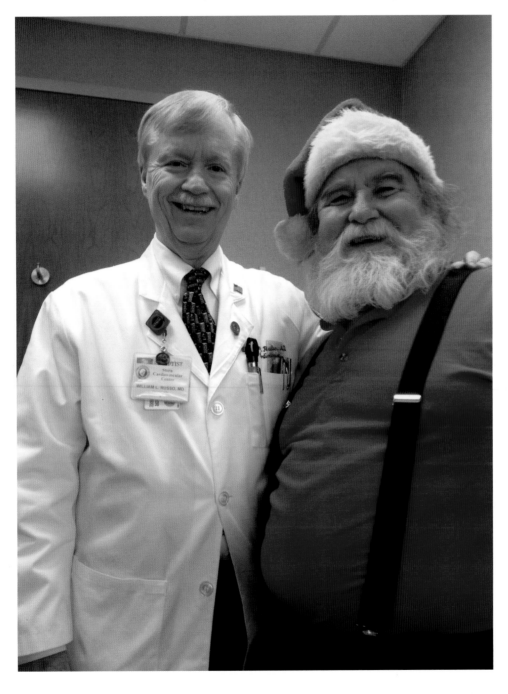

▲ Dr. William Russo with Santa

Photo thanks to Stern Cardio

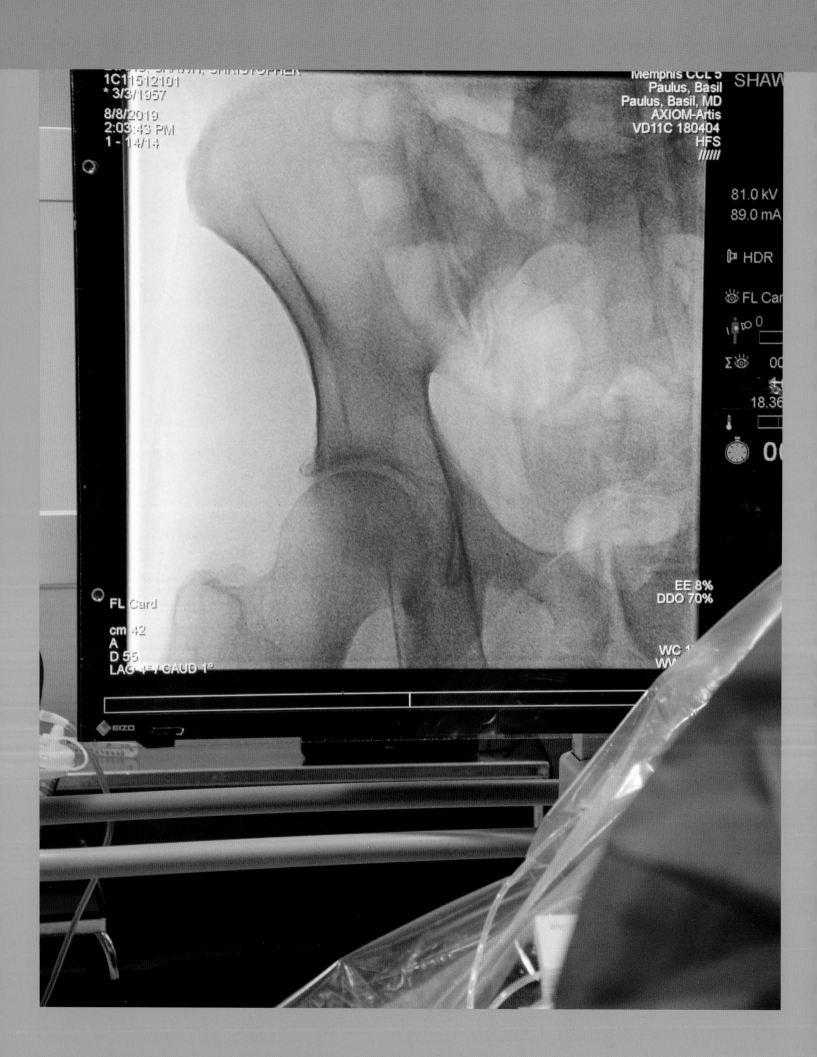

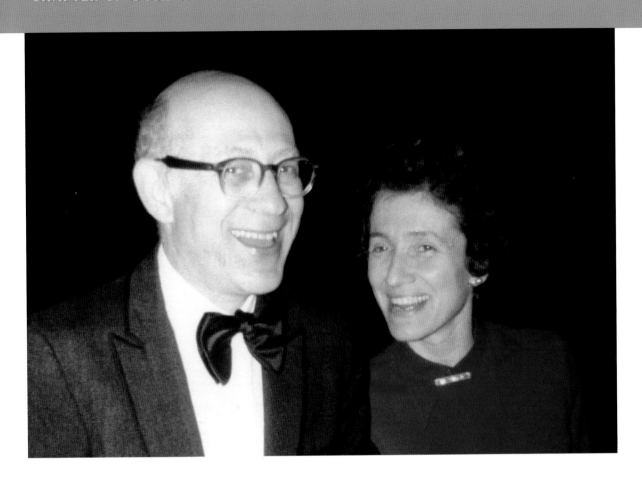

◀ Tom and Harriet Stern
Photo thanks to David Stern

WITHIN ALL OF MEDICINE, THE 1980S ARE CONSIDERED TO BE A HISTORIC DE-CADE FOR CARDIOLOGY; THE HARD-FOUGHT MOMENT WHEN STEADY IM-PROVEMENTS IN DIAGNOSTIC IMAGING, REFINED OVER THE COURSE OF DE-CADES, COULD BE SUPPORTED BY ACUTE INTERVENTIONS. ACE INHIBITORS APPEARED EARLY ON. THROMBOLYTIC MEDICATIONS WERE SO WIDELY AND ENTHUSIASTICAL-LY ADOPTED, SOME SCHOLARS REFER TO THE 1980S AS THE "THROMBOLYTIC ERA."

Certainly, Andreas Gruentzig's alternative, less-invasive proce-dure—which would be dubbed percutaneous transluminal coro-nary angioplasty, or PTCA—rev-olutionized the treatment of coro-nary artery disease. As McFarland and Pitts wrote: "In adults, PTCA via balloon-tipped catheter essen-tially defined the overlap between diagnosis and intervention because expanding the balloon could treat as well as identify blockages in the coronary arteries."

"When I started, we didn't treat heart attacks, just the complica-tions. But shortly after joining, clot-busting drugs, balloons to open up arteries . . . a much more scientific basis for treating things came into use." —Frank McGrew, M.D., Director of Clinical Research, Stern Cardiovascular Foundation

By the mid-1980s, McFarland and Pitts report, Memphis cardiologists performed balloon treatments and bypass surgeries in equal number. In 1986, a treat-ment to rival PTCA appeared: the intracoronary stent. The authors note that the treatment was "quickly adopted at major hospitals . . . employed by inter-ventional cardiologists from the Stern Clinic, the Memphis Heart Clinic and others." In 1985, Stern launched its transplant program, another front-running move within the region.

As the Stern Clinic—a colloquial name for the Cardiology Group of Memphis—tested breakthrough technologies on the front lines, staff members pioneered critical support programs in the back office. While Tom Stern provided the vision, Judy Jackson built the practice's first in-house clinical lab, for example. But first, CGoM would hire its first licensed nurses. The year was 1980.

The Vanguard of Nurses

"It takes a lot of critical thinking, compassion and time to train to be a Stern Cardiovascular nurse. But if you want to make a difference and want a home, you're going to be rewarded." —Pamela Burks, Director of Nursing, Stern Cardiovascular Foundation

As registered nurses in Baptist's coronary care unit, Kathy Baker (now Kathy Gwinn) and Patty Hatcher had been acquainted with, nay, working with CGoM physicians, for quite some time. In fact, when talk of hiring nurses circulated around the office in the decade prior, David Holloway conducted what was akin to a discovery interview with Kathy, aimed at exploring how nurses might fit into the practice.

About a year later, Kathy received a call from Patty. While working together on the coronary floor of the hospital, Frank McGrew had asked Patty if she and Kathy would like to come to work as cardiology nurses at his practice. When Randy Meeks finished her training, she joined them. The Cardiology Group of Memphis had its first team of registered nurses.

Despite the doctors' readiness to staff nurses, the process of defin-ing the nurses' role was a work in progress. In the beginning, every day was an opportunity to add a new job responsibility and refine the working relationship. Patty Hatcher describes how the role took shape:

"Initially, we answered the phone and made rounds with doctors, pulling charts. But as time went on, we started gathering infor-mation, starting chart notes and answering patient calls. We weren't as specialized then, and we could get involved in almost anything. Drs. McGrew and Salky were involved in research projects, and we got to be involved with those. All of the doctors were such wonderful teachers. They taught me things as a young nurse about cardiology, the physiology behind things, how to take care of people ... they didn't hesitate to share what they knew with the people around them."

As modeled by physicians in the practice, CGoM nurses placed a high value on patient relation-ships. "We made a connection with patients [and] gave doctors time to do things you needed to be more educated to do. Other times we gave doctors more time to spend with their patients. I think one of our biggest roles was serv-ing as a liaison between patients, nurses, doctors, secretaries and hospitals," Kathy remembers.

David Stern shares a similar sen-timent when recalling his father's working relationship with Randy Meeks. "They were able to see 45 patients on a Saturday morning mostly because of the closeness with which he and Randy worked, and knowing the patients. That made them both enormously efficient," David explains.

When Patty reflects on the time when the role of nurses at Stern was less defined, there's a smile in her voice. "It didn't take long for them to figure out what to do with us," she says. Nor did they ever look back: At the end of the decade, the practice would staff 26 nurses for 13 doctors. Leading into 2020, that number has climbed to 80 nurses—85, counting PRNs—allowing each doctor at least one nurse and building sufficient staffing for Stern Cardiovascular Foundation's ancillary services, such as the Anticoagulation and Pacer Clinics.

The integration of nurses is a topic that David Holloway, too, touched on as he detailed the practice's evolution. "When the early guys were practicing, we didn't have nurses. We took our own call. I would come home, get in bed, get a call, get right out of bed and go back to the hospital. We were up all night working our tails off. That changed over the years to where we rarely have to go out at night and we don't get phone calls because nurses take the calls at night and only relay to the doctor if there's an emergency," David explains.

Taking Care of Business

In the 1980s, CGoM would also make a fundamental change in its business administration—a change that would bolster the group's confidence to grow in size and offering.

Dan Caldwell was working in corporate finance for Memphis' Schering-Plough when his friend Joe Samaha passed along a tip: The Cardiology Group of Memphis was looking to hire an administrator with a background in business. Dan Caldwell had an MBA in finance but no interest, as he puts it, in "managing a doctor's office." Nonetheless, Dan had breakfast with some of the group's senior ranks. "The questions they were asking, I was answering very honestly—rather than answering in ways they wanted to hear," Dan remembers. If his honesty was a tactic to take himself out of the running, it didn't work. "They liked it, and called me the next day," Dan says.

Dan accepted the role of Executive Director, CGoM's senior administrative role, in 1987. For the first time in its history, the group had a business administrator whose experience went beyond managing a practice and extended to creating financial analysis and projections. Yet for all of the expertise Dan brought to the group, he's quick to share, "I can't tell you how much I learned from Tom Stern about balancing all these things: being attuned to the business—making good business decisions—while caring about people, too."

It was with this worldview that Dan got to work analyzing the feasibility of new projects, which included developing comprehensive financial statements and strategic planning. His first project revealed itself immediately: At the time Dan went to work for CGoM, physician schedules were booked four to six months ahead. Relying on the honesty that had landed him in his new role, Dan told the group that it was losing patients. "When patients can't see you, you know that they're calling competitors," he told them, following up with a plan to overhaul physician schedules. Existing patient visits would be shortened

slightly to create room—and the additional time needed—for new patient visits. "Volumes went up 20 to 30 percent just with our existing doctors," Dan reports, though the group knew it needed to push for more. "We really needed to expand the group, but hiring a new cardiologist takes an investment," says Dan. He developed financial models detailing the impact of growing the staff and adding offices. "It gave the decision-makers more comfort and confidence to grow," Dan reports.

If the practice initially required growth for survival, it would soon rely on growth to fuel ancillary initiatives. Dan explains how the practice worked toward formalizing and growing its outreach efforts:

"It was one of those things where you had to look deeper than just the clinic itself. If you just look at the revenue of the [outreach] clinic and the expense to go there, it doesn't look very good: You're going to send a cardiologist, a nurse and a medical assistant to this little clinic once a week and take the full day to see 20 or 30 patients, but we won't have diagnostics and we have to pay rent. But, if you're going to be there once a week, the local medical community thinks about you when they see a patient with a heart problem. When someone urgent can't wait, they'll send them to you in Memphis. When they get a patient with chest pain, they start calling your cardiologist on call. The 20 or 30 patients you see once a week turns into 150 or 200 patients."

After a time, Dan conducted a zip code analysis to measure the impact of CGoM's growing out-

reach efforts. "Before the outreach clinics, we were seeing 80 percent of patients from Shelby County. After the outreach clinics, we were seeing 40 percent from Shelby County and 60 percent from surrounding counties further away," he reports. The analysis confirmed Dan's original hypothesis: Outreach would turn CGoM from a local cardiology practice to a regional resource.

There's one more truth Dan relates in his final analysis: The refinement of CGoM's outreach efforts began with a baseline established by Tom Stern. "We learned from what he was doing," Dan recalls, suggesting something beyond the years of clinical outreach experience Tom had to share. Dan was deeply impressed by the way Tom interacted with local physicians:

"As brilliant as he was, he was such a great listener and so respectful of what local physicians were doing. He listened a lot, affirmed them a lot, expressed his respect for what they were doing; it was more along the lines of, 'I'm here to help. What can I do?' What I was struck by was that that was exactly the right approach to take. Nobody had to tell them he was a brilliant cardiologist, it's that mutual respect he developed with people."

It was a lesson Dan would call on to develop mutually respectful relationships with hospital administrators as part of CGoM's outreach efforts. If an administrator ever needed reassurance, Dan would personally call on them. He would establish that CGoM was there to step in when a patient needed cardiology services the hospital couldn't provide—and that CGoM would send the pa-

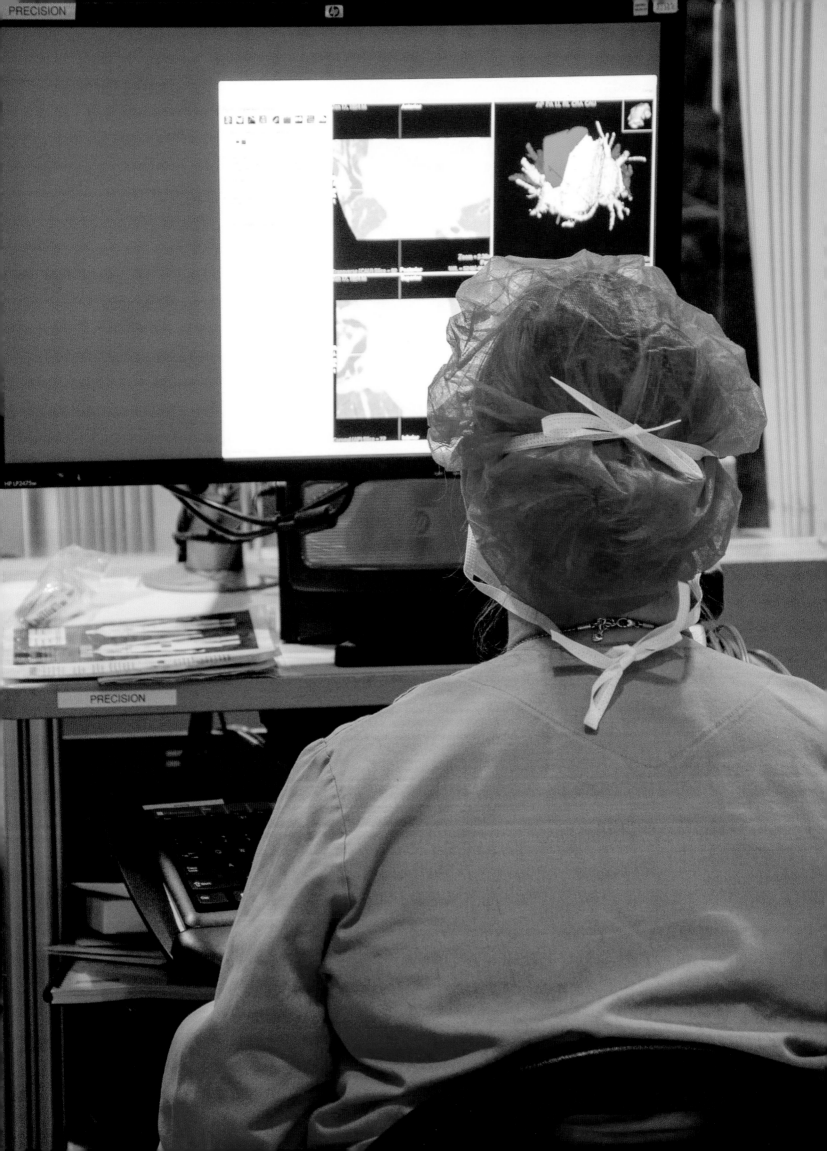

tient right back to the hometown hospital when the patient needed services outside of cardiology. "We were getting patients back consistently," Dan reports, and trust built between CGoM and the hospitals in its outreach areas.

The success of yet another program built confidence—and aligned with the goals—of CGoM's management team. "They wanted to see the practice grow into more of what they were capable of doing," Dan recalls. Once solidly on a path toward growth, the practice was ready to look at adding services.

At the time—the late 1980s—Dan recalls:

"Nuclear imaging was getting busier and busier. We were in an office building across from the hospital attached by a tunnel. We sent patients over to Baptist for nuclear imaging, but we wanted to get info on the patient sooner—we were sometimes waiting 30 or 60 days. Then one day it occurred to some of us that maybe we should look at [investing in] our own imaging."

Dan considered other cardiology clinics across the country that had run with the same thought. The benefits were evident: a dramatically shortened turnaround time for test results and even a little profit for the practice. Still, it would be the biggest single investment CGoM had ever made. "When you say, 'We're going to invest half-a-million dollars in something' in a group that was only six or seven cardiologists, that was quite a scary thing," Dan readily admits. But he followed up with a strong analysis detailing what insurance would cover; how many tests a day would consti-

tute break-even; cost and revenue breakdowns. As with the financial modeling Dan had shared relevant to the hiring of new physicians, his analysis gave the group confidence. "They decided to do it and it turned out to be a great success for patient care," Dan asserts.

As the group and its offerings grew, so did the need to manage its day-to-day operations more efficiently. Dan remembers reading an article about an architecture firm in Florida that was advocating for a pod concept in healthcare practice design. Whereas traditional design placed exam rooms off of long hallways, inconvenient to areas where nurses and medical assistants worked, the pod concept centered those areas around the exam rooms. "We were starting to think about designing new offices, so I went over the pod concept with the doctors. They agreed that it was a much more efficient way to operate," Dan remembers, and the discovery process officially began. "We visited a clinic in Charlotte, North Carolina, that had just finished designing their clinic that way," Dan recalls. Then, CGoM hired the firm from the article Dan had read to design two of its offices: first, the downtown medical center; not long after, CGoM's Baptist East location. "That's the way most offices are still designed and we were innovative in building out our clinics in a pod concept at that time," Dan says.

Outreach

"We encouraged each other in the direction of covering more communities than just Memphis, because we realized that our patient base wasn't just Memphis. People were driving hundreds of miles to get here because Memphis was

a city that had big hospitals that could take care of everybody. But driving hundreds of miles was not going to be a sustainable model. Outreach became a huge effort."
—Debbie Eddlestone, CEO, Stern Cardiovascular Foundation

You could say that Stern Cardiovascular Foundation's emphasis on outreach began with Neuton Stern, who practiced in an era when house calls were standard. Becky Conner, Administrative Assistant to Drs. David Holloway and Eric Johnson, recently received a modern-day reminder of the practice's age-old way of doing business: At an appointment with her doctor, Conner mentioned that she was on her way to the celebration of William Russo's retirement and David Holloway's 50th anniversary with Stern. Becky's doctor shared that her own grandfather had been a patient of Neuton Stern. Going through her grandfather's effects, the doctor found an invoice issued by Neuton Stern for a house call in Tunica. "When I told Dr. Holloway," Becky notes, "he said they all used to make house calls when he first started with them."

In terms of pure outreach, however, Tom Stern led the way. As some stories tell it, he began developing relationships with doctors in Forrest City, Arkansas, when he moonlit in the area as a resident. (His mother, Beatrice, was a native of Paragould, Arkansas, and it has also been said that Neuton gave talks in the area.) Whatever the case, Tom committed to the region. In time, he added Wynne, Arkansas, to his rotation, seeing patients in Wynne in the morning and Forrest City in the afternoon on his designated outreach day.

Also in time, the group designated outreach nurses to travel with practice doctors to their adopted outreach clinics. This explains why Randy Meeks didn't accompany Tom on his outreach missions initially. That changed the last few years before Tom's death.

"I would pick him up at his house and it would take about an hour and 15 minutes to get over there. I'd call new patients the night before and get their medical histories and he would read them on the way. Then on the way back, he'd spend the time dictating," Randy remembers. Between drives, the schedule was demanding. "In Memphis, Dr. Stern was trying to limit the number of patients he had a day and to limit new patients to one a day," Randy explains, continuing, "but when we went to Forrest City, there were no limits. That list would be so long and he didn't tell anybody 'no.' We'd see eight to 12 new patients a day—more than that considering existing patients."

As the biggest city in the Mississippi Delta region, Memphis was uniquely positioned to dispatch highly qualified physicians to surrounding underserved areas. The populations of proximate rural and feeder cities already considered Memphis their "local" medical hub. Into this context, CGoM dispatched additional physicians, weaving the first threads of its outreach network.

Jan Turner and Sharon Goldstein collaborated on a program in Ripley, Tennessee. Sharon shares this recollection of their earliest days:

"We'd go from this cosmopolitan setting [in Memphis] to being the man with the medicine bag.

I was the only person who went with Jan. I'd do everything from scheduling the appointments to collecting the payments. So many people in that small area wouldn't go see anybody else; they would be standing in line to see 'Dr. T' on the Tuesdays that we would go there. We had a little bitty room in a hospital with a portable EKG and we would just take care of people. It got us so involved with the small communities, with farmers . . . people would bring us Ripley tomatoes in payment." Jan adds, "I went there until I retired, and was fortunate to have some really good primary care physicians out there."

Similarly, David Holloway reached out to Savannah, Tennessee, and Ripley, Mississippi. While David no longer travels to his outreach communities, he reports, "I still see patients every day from those areas. I guess they liked me."

Frank McGrew helped extend CGoM's outreach to Clarksdale, Mississippi. "That area of the United States was one of the poorest around. These were very underserved people," he explains. Drawing on relationships he had cultivated over the years with primary care physicians in the area, and expanding his network through referrals and acquaintances made at hospital-based seminars and regional meetings, Frank built a caseload. Through the years, CGoM's outreach grew from a mobile trailer to an office space within the hospital itself. Of the program, Frank is most proud of the rare level of care he was able to bring to the community, reminiscing, "We were able to put a lot of patients into clinical trials so they were able to receive cutting-edge care."

William Russo, accompanied by Pamela Burks, also participated in the practice's outreach to Mississippi. Pamela remembers that after one particularly long day, rather than returning immediately to the city, the pair took a detour. "Dr. Russo wanted to stop by a patient's home who was in hospice there. The family appreciated that so much and for me, it was a teaching moment about compassion. That's when I knew I had my [professional] home—I wanted to be a part of that," Pamela shares.

In time, Steven Gubin would reach out to Hayti, Missouri, while Drs. Todd Edwards and Amit Malhotra deepened the practice's engagement in Mississippi.

Despite living in Germantown, Tennessee, Amit Malhotra felt a mandate to practice in the Mississippi Delta. His choice was influenced by observations, not unlike those of his colleagues, of an area poorly served: populated with patients who lacked an understanding of, and access to, care; a population limited by factors other patients might take for granted—such as transportation challenges. How does a physician overcome such odds? According to Amit, you build a bridge. It starts with building relationships with physicians in smaller hospitals. But the outreach process is equally about building relationships with patients. And in the Mississippi Delta, that can mean providing care regardless of a patient's ability to pay, availing patients of assistance and insurance options—and connecting them to the program that best fits their needs. "Nobody is refused care. We work with patients and the Baptist Memorial

Health Care Foundation," Amit explains, referring to Baptist's non-profit initiative to provide financial assistance to uninsured, and underinsured, patients. "We have such a terrible system for people who don't have access [to healthcare]. Critically sick patients without access get shunted from one place to another; a lot of places will not see you unless you have proof of insurance, especially in an outpatient setting. Sometimes it takes a personal effort to write to a state senator to facilitate getting appropriate help: getting them onto the state medical assistance program or Affordable Care. We have processes where we streamline all of that," Amit explains.

"We've made a policy of not caring who's coming from where. If it's a critically sick patient who's been refused elsewhere, we don't care about that. We just take care of them." —Amit Malhotra, M.D., Stern Cardiovascular Foundation

After the bridge is built, Amit continues, the goal is to "create channels so that patients get specialized care in the big hospitals. Then they go back to their communities. And we're right there to monitor them as part of our outreach, rather than the patient going back and forth." The effect? "Just sitting in the office and having people call you is one thing. But if you do outreach and take care of them on an ongoing basis, then bring them back for specialized care, it will lead to less admissions, [increased] longevity and continuity of care in concert with local providers," Amit asserts.

While Debbie reports that Stern Cardiovascular Foundation's current presence in Mississippi is almost as great as its presence in Memphis, she notes that the group's outreach efforts are even wider in scope:

"When we took on Dr. Richard Gordon in 2010, he had already created outreach locations himself as a sole practitioner. He really knew how to do it and how to get into the communities that had the greatest need," Debbie says. Richard sees patients at Stern's outreach facilities in Oakland and Ripley, Tennessee. Meanwhile, Louis Caruso, M.D., has established Stern outreach outposts in Huntingdon and Union City, Tennessee (Union City has since evolved into a physical location for the group). In its centennial year, Stern Cardiovascular Foundation maintains nine outreach locations across Arkansas, Mississippi and Tennessee:

Arkansas: West Memphis

Mississippi: Columbus, Corinth, New Albany

Tennessee: Halls, Huntingdon, Midtown Memphis, Oakland, Ripley

The Clinical Lab

When Judy Jackson joined the Cardiology Group of Memphis around 1985, the group performed a small amount of testing in-house, but outsourced the majority. As Judy remembers: "The few tests they had weren't challenging for me, but it was a change from the hospital schedule I'd been working. Then Dr. Stern called me in and that was a real challenge."

As it turns out, Tom had learned of Judy's laboratory background. Judy recalls of their conversation, "Dr. Stern had thought about opening a lab for our patients and doctors so we could get test results back more quickly. But he didn't know how to go about it and asked if I could help him. He said if I could get the information on the equipment, he could find some space." Tom delivered on his end and Judy set to work bringing in everything from water and electricity to countertops and, finally, equipment. The Cardiology Group of Memphis Clinical Lab opened in February 1987.

Judy was the lab's only employee for a time. The first person hired to help her didn't last. "It was overwhelming. We would have to work late and stay until we finished," Judy remembers. That spring, Judy's niece, Pam Glover, completed school and joined her aunt in the lab. "Then it was the two of us working late and staying until we finished," Judy laughs, adding, "It was a labor of love and it was an opportunity."

Pam shared her memories of those formative years:

"We brought an analyzer in and did chemistries and CBCs in-house that the group had never done before. We had students who would come rotate through from the lab program. Otherwise it was just the two of us and we were the lab, with Dr. Stern as our lab director."

"The lab was Dr. Stern's passion—and treating patients like family," says Pam Glover. She explains Tom's approach to the lab as continual inquiry, based on the question: "What can we do for patients to keep them from getting as sick?" Since Tom's curiosity was as persistent as his interest in research, that combination informed every stage of the growth of CGoM's Clinical Lab.

Having been involved nearly from the beginning, Pam recaps key milestones:

Leading in technology: "Whatever new was on the horizon, [Dr. Stern] would say, 'Let's find out about this,' and he'd already have done half the research or more," Pam recalls fondly. In fact, Tom was one of the first people in Memphis to do proton INR recording. Pam remembers Tom asserting that the leading-edge protocol would become the new standard, protecting the integrity of recordings from variations in analyzers and reagents. After Tom positioned his lab as first to market, Pam remembers, "Hospitals would call us asking us how we were doing it." Judy adds, "We helped those hospitals and clinics set their programs up."

Of course, this wasn't the only time that Tom would position his lab ahead of the curve. "He was really good about anything that our lab needed. If we started sending out a bunch of tests, he would check into it and see if it was feasible for us to bring it in-house," Pam says. Tom's "early adopter" approach became fundamental to the lab's mission, even as he was compelled to step back. "About a year before he died, he finally turned the lab over. But he was still up on everything. I wished he'd stop reading all the articles because every time he did, he'd say, 'Let's try this!'" Pam says, lightheartedly. In all seriousness, she shares, "Dr. Stern made me want to learn and do better. It was an honor to work with him and it's an honor to still work here and be able to honor his legacy."

What does that legacy look like today? Pam reports: "We've really

come a long way. We do more clinical work in our lab than some hospitals; our proton analyzer is a smaller version of the instrument used on campus at Baptist. With Baptist being our hospital, we all wanted that integrity," Pam explains, noting that the setup allows Stern to "maintain great results."

Leading the standard: Just as Tom extended his and his lab's help to other hospital and clinic labs—including setting up normal values for Le Bonheur Children's Hospital—he remained focused on the greater good. As Judy recalls:

"He wanted our reference lab to flag cholesterol at 200 instead of 300 because he thought 300 was too high. He wanted me to call our reference lab and tell them to flag them. Their reaction was, 'You want us to change that?' and I said, 'That's what Dr. Stern would like.' They said, 'We'll talk about it in our board meeting and let you know.' After a couple weeks, they sent our reports back flagged at 200. When I told Dr. Stern that the lab was going to flag our cholesterol at 200, he said, 'Are they just going to do our patients? That's not good enough. They have to do everybody's patients. You go back and call them.' I called back and they started flagging everybody's. No one else in the whole tri-state area was doing that. It was probably another six months before national labs started flagging [at that level]. Now it's a national standard."

Similarly, Judy remembers Tom specifying that his lab's lipids should match those of the National Lipid Foundation. "Even though it wasn't required, we went

over and above because patient care and quality were so important to him. It wasn't enough to meet the status quo. We set higher standards because we were Stern. That made us who we were," Judy says.

Leading in quality: Committing to operating on the leading edge, and on par with partner hospitals, also sets Stern's clinical lab up to achieve the most elite accreditations. "Before it was required, we chose to go for national accreditation," Judy explains. Though it was her decision to make, she credits Tom for the motivation. "He inspired you to set your goals high. That's the way he was and you wanted to do everything the best you could, too," she shares.

The lab earned its first national accreditation through the Commission on Office Laboratory Accreditation (COLA) in 1992. In its most recent audit (2017), the lab scored 100 percent. Pam describes the process as, "300 questions on anything. They can ask over [the course of] six to eight hours and look at two years' worth of data." After receiving its perfect score, Stern's Clinical Lab was contacted by the Tennessee board. "They wanted to check behind the COLA auditor because it's so rare to get a 100 percent," Pam remembers with pride. "We made 100 percent with the state also," she adds.

Advocating for prevention: "Dr. Stern's philosophy is carried forward now by initiatives like twice-monthly screenings," Pam says, describing Stern's routine practice of inviting the public in for preventive assessment. Twice a month, 11 months of the year, staff members representing various departments work into the evening to administer the program. Existing and new patients are welcome, and sometimes nearly 30 will fill the schedule. They rotate between stations, each one equipped to perform a different diagnostic test. The lab processes the test results the following day and releases them to Steven Gubin, who creates an individualized follow-up letter for each participant. Pam likes to think of these as tips to keep participants from becoming patients.

"It makes me feel good to go to work every day because I'm going to be able to help a doctor help a patient." —Pam Glover, Clinical Lab Manager, Stern Cardiovascular Foundation

Providing a one-stop shop: The existence of Stern's lab allows a patient to receive a physician consult, diagnostic procedures, lab services and prescription fulfillment all in the same visit. Making the patient experience even smoother, Pam reports, "hospitals will even take our results (within two-and-a-half weeks) so patients don't have to get tests redone . . . they know our results are accurate."

Prioritizing personalized care: "We do close to 250 samples a day from five Stern locations and we treat every sample like there's a person behind it," Pam asserts. Now as Clinical Lab Manager, following Judy's retirement in 2016 after 33 years in the post, Pam leads a lab team of five in a manner wholly inspired by Tom Stern: "We want to treat you, our patient, like it's just you and me," she says.

WALKING THE WALK

Of Tom Stern, Randy Meeks says, "He practiced what he preached." He didn't smoke. He limited his consumption of red meat. He knew his cholesterol numbers. And those who worked with him saw Tom take active measures to keep his own blood pressure down. "He and Harriet walked every night; he came down to exercise in the gym three to four times a week," Randy recalls. As David Stern remembers, every day his father walked into the office, "he would step on the scale. Randy used to put her foot on the scale just to mess with him," David relays fondly.

Nancy Cummings shares a remembrance here, too. "When I became a nurse, the first time I was going to round with Dr. Stern, we get over to the old Baptist Hospital. The cardiac floors were 14 and 15. We get to the elevator and he walks to the stairs and says, 'Nancy, you are welcome to take the elevator.' He always took the stairs," Nancy says. David was another witness. "When I started medical school, my father let me come on rounds with him. He was well-known for taking the stairs, much to the chagrin of the residents and med students," David notes.

Another time, Nancy and Tom had traveled to Columbia, South Carolina, to study how another practice was managing its medical records. Nancy, who was at the time preparing for her Boards of Nursing, sat to study during a layover. Again, Tom graciously gave her an out: "He said, 'Now Nancy, I'm going to be walking if you want to walk with me.' And I would look up and he walked

that airport like he was in a hurry to get to a flight—all the way up until it was time for us to board, " she remembers.

Randy adds that, "Dr. Stern ate the way he told his patients to eat—though he absolutely loved barbecue." And once, on an outing to the Racquet Club, he even tried a Pronto Pup, Memphis' own golden-fried hotdog on a stick. Randy ordered one first and Tom had to ask her what it was. After trying his own, he pronounced, "That Pronto Pup was awful."

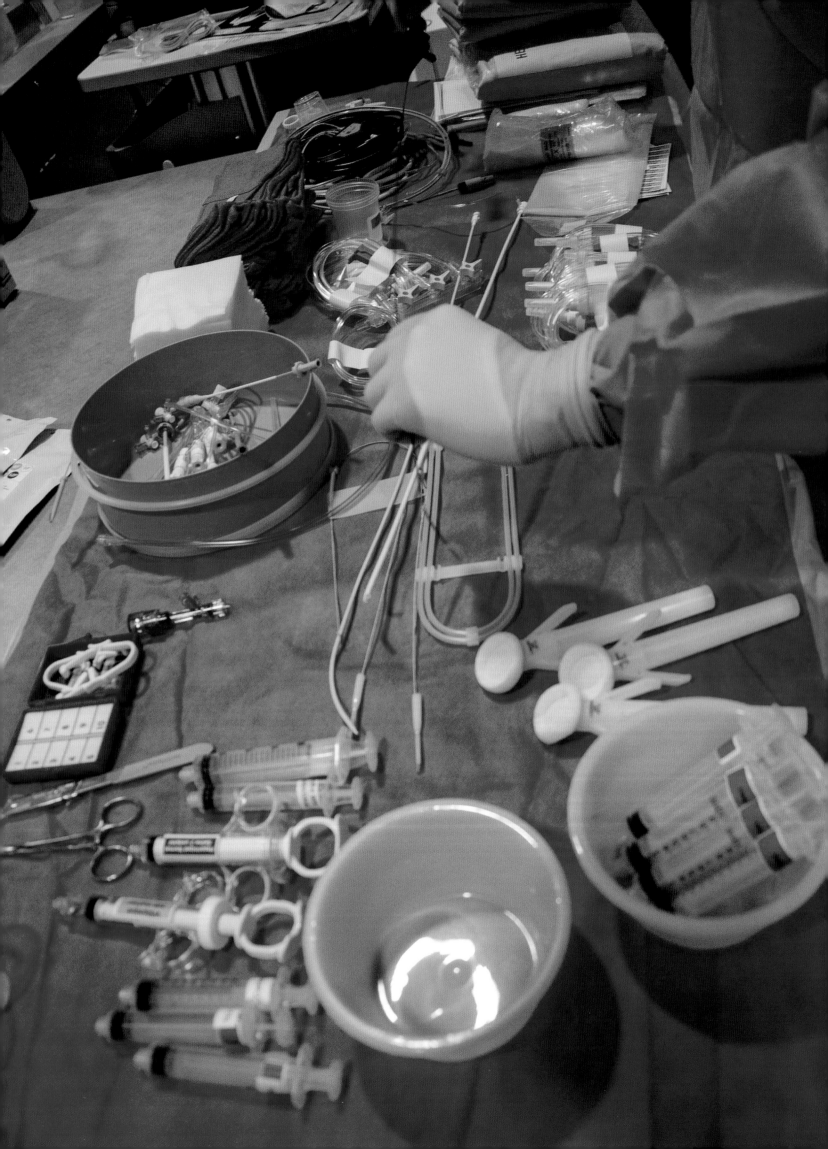

Reading this chapter, it's easy to get swept up in the advancements of the decade, from universal strides in cardiology to expansion within the microcosm of Stern. What makes the headlines of the era even more compelling, however, is their backstory: a series of challenges that paints the decade's highs in stark relief.

The challenges arose when a new computer system failed, crippling the practice's ability to collect payments. But the threat of insolvency proved an impetus. "It was a turning point," remembers David Holloway, and the steps toward recovery that it inspired combined methodical business strategy with pure passion.

David Holloway explains how the practice's financial recovery was kickstarted. "We took equal salaries below what we could have made. That said a lot about the doctors in this group," he says. Then a loan was secured from

First Tennessee Bank. These acts weren't merely a matter of dollars and cents: Employees on the inside track remember Dr. Holloway working tirelessly to secure the trust of his colleagues, and of the bank, in the practice.

To ensure long-term solvency, outsiders were recruited to manage the business aspects of the practice, and those individuals recruited others in turn. Marty Grusin, a Memphis attorney, was among them. Marty recruited a friend with experience in education and healthcare, Dr. Fred Klyman, to help him manage the practice.

Together, they helped recruit Debbie Eddlestone as Director of the Business Office. Dan Caldwell, who had moved on from the practice, returned to ensure that all hands were on deck.

Like Dan Caldwell's job interview with Stern a decade prior, Debbie Eddlestone's 1997 interview was marked by straight talk. "I asked her if she knew what it means to see the rocks at the bottom of the pond," David Holloway remembers. "And she really knew how to collect money," he soon learned. Marty too credits Debbie, along with Fred Klyman and Stern's

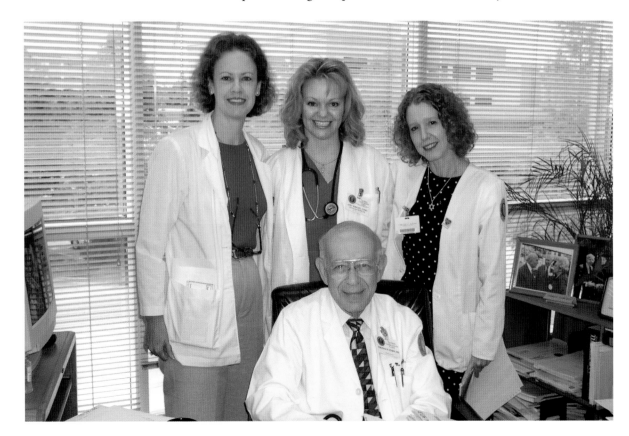

◀◀ The Operating Room
Photo by Stephanie Norwood

◀ Randy Meeks, Amy Wright, Elissa Fine, and Tom Stern
Photo thanks to Randy Meeks

current-day CFO Melissa Reaves, for laying the groundwork for the group's long-term financial success. "Tom Stern built this institution into a group of great doctors. The contribution that Fred, Debbie and Melissa made was to organize those great doctors into an independent institution that could satisfy the needs of the patients as well as the doctors," Marty explains.

With this goal achieved, the practice could exercise freedom to pursue growth initiatives. Marty Grusin chronicled how different financing was arranged with the bank to allow for the expansion of Stern's staff, physical footprint and other capabilities you'll read about in this chapter. All the while, Marty recalls, Drs. Stern and Holloway were facilitating the practice's rehabilitation in their own way: bringing the individual members of their group together. As the practice overcame the challenges of the late 1990s, it was natural that Stern physicians would have differing theories regarding how to move the group forward. "You had talented people with their own thoughts on what to do, but you had to keep them going in the same direction. Drs. Holloways and Stern managed that. They were not only doctors, they were statesmen," Marty asserts.

WELCOME, STEVEN GUBIN

Steven Gubin had always had ties to Memphis. His grandfather, a U.S. Army doctor, came to Memphis from New York following World War II to run the outpatient center at the old VA hospital. Steven's father was a doctor too, but when he developed heart disease, he saw Tom Stern. It

was a familiar relationship. "Tom I knew well," Steven shares, adding, "He took care of my family when I was a kid."

While Steven stayed in Memphis for medical school, he left for several years to train—a period that took him from the National Institutes of Health in Bethesda, Maryland, to China to Penn State's Hershey Medical Center. "When I finished my training, I came back to Memphis," Steven shares, adding, "I looked around a lot first and got offers, but a lot of things attracted me to the offer here. My dad was practicing in Missouri and the group was really big on outreach. It gave me an opportunity: For 15 years, I went to work in the same hospital as my dad. I'd go every week and drive two hours one way."

Back at CGoM's main office in Memphis, Steven recalls what it was like settling in:

"Dr. Stern always believed that people should sub-specialize. In some cardiology groups, everybody does everything. But in this group, it was more like a private practice where everyone specialized. I cath'd when I came here, but I never cath'd once I got here because there were docs who were experts in that. I did the ultrasounds and nuclear stress tests, so I got to specialize in that area. The guys who did the caths were sending stuff to us to do nuclear echos; if we had something abnormal, we'd send it to them."

Steven's specialty was, in fact, trans-esophogal echocardiography, one of the many advancements in diagnostics that surfaced in the 1990s. "It was just coming out then, so I was able to add something new to the group that no

one else was doing. That was nice," he shares.

"My relationship with Stern came with Tommy [Dr. Tom Stern], who was my cardiologist. When Dr. Stern took ill, he [called] me and told me he would have to stop practicing and wanted to recommend Steve Gubin. As to Steve, he is highly respected, loved by all of his patients and admired." —Jack Belz, Chairman and CEO of Belz Enterprises

NUCLEAR CARDIOLOGY

Scot Feury shared Steven Gubin's interest in nuclear imaging, joining the practice two months later. Scot had completed his schooling and worked at Baptist, including a stint with John F. Rockett, M.D., the world-renowned nuclear physician who directed the Nuclear Medicine Division of Baptist's Radiology Department. The division's lead technologist—Scot's direct supervisor—was Jimmy Smith. Around 1989, Scot remembers, Jimmy left. "He left after being in charge of one of the busiest departments in one of the largest hospitals in the Southeast," Scot says. So where did Jimmy go? "To work for the Cardiology Group of Memphis right across the street," Scot responds, painting a picture of those late-1980s days, before the proliferation of sleek centers built to perform outpatient procedures: "There was such a backlog for the Cardiology Group of Memphis to get their patients' nuclear cardiology studies. Whether pre-op or pre-discharge, patients were having to stay in the hospital for days to get these tests done," Scot recalls.

Scot acknowledges that length of stay has always been a hot topic.

But as with so many decisions in the history of CGoM, patient care and quality were top of mind. "This was one of the first groups to hire a nuclear medicine technician. The primary reason was so patients could have the tests done in the group's office," Scot says. That was Jimmy Smith's charge: building the group's in-house nuclear imaging capacity downtown. In 1991, Scot got the call from Jimmy. "He asked, 'What would it take for you to come and have a camera at our Baptist East location?' They could see that everything was starting to move east," Scot noted, and accepted the invitation to open CGoM's second nuclear imaging site, with one camera and a room not much bigger than a closet. For patients, the change was drastic: In place of overnight or multi-day inpatient stays, "Patients could go through a tunnel that connected the hospital to our office. We performed the nuclear studies in our office, and our doctors would read them," Scot explains.

Steven Gubin was given responsibility for the group's Nuclear Cardiology Department, and its scope grew. It wasn't just that CGoM was one of the first groups to advance nuclear medicine in Memphis—the group built the very path forward. As Scot notes, "We were able to try all the new reagents from the pharmacy and any new testing that was being put out for the heart. Our office was one of the first in Memphis to receive accreditation from the Intersocietal Accreditation Commission (IAC)." The fact that CGoM doctors were reading their own nuclear study test results "was a bold step back then," Scot recalls. It still isn't the norm, and yet about half of Stern's present-day staff are nuclear readers who undergo a special preceptorship and achieve certification through the American Board of Nuclear Medicine.

For Scot, now Nuclear Cardiology Supervisor for Stern and Baptist, being first-to-market in nuclear imaging in Memphis was never about being first in and of itself— it's always been about the patients. Because the diagnostic phase can be among a patient's earliest, and most fraught, interactions with any practice, Scot trains his staff of 15 to anticipate patient anxiety and provide a personal level of comfort. "We work with patients to help them understand why we're doing what we're doing," he explains, and that's just the start. "There is redundant equipment, and offerings, at some Stern locations and hospitals, so patients can decide what's more convenient. They can have the procedure done with Stern or with the hospital; it's all charged the same way if it's a Stern or Baptist location," Scot explains. In addition, the hospital and Stern have partnered on initiatives such as the low-risk chest pain protocol. Under the protocol, patients who present at a Baptist emergency room with chest pain, but prove to be otherwise low-risk on an evidence-based scale, avoid routine hospitalization. Instead, as Scot explains, "They leave under the premise that they're going to come to Stern and have a treadmill test [or the equivalent] done within 48 hours. It keeps them from staying overnight."

Not only a matter of convenience, the Stern-Baptist collaboration impacts quality of care. For Scot, it's the difference between seeing patients once or twice as a tech working in a hospital and seeing the same patients every year or two: "You can follow patients so much closer. You get involved with their care and see the effects that everyone on our team has on these patients' lives. I'm just a small part but I can see it, following a patient from my test to a catheter test through a bypass or pacemaker procedure," he shares.

ADVANCES IN INTERVENTIONAL CARDIOLOGY

As techniques and devices including, but not limited to, imaging innovated in the 1990s, so did physician training. David Wolford had just completed a fellowship in cardiology at the University of Tennessee at Memphis in 1995 when the American College of Cardiology announced a change: an additional year of training would now be required for rising interventional cardiologists. In fact, David would become the very first interventional cardiologist trained at the University of Tennessee. In 1996, he joined CGoM.

Of those early days, David recalls:

"We were doing rotational, directional and laser atherectomy, new stenting procedures and interventional ultrasound. Our devices that had been very large, and that required large incisions and manual compression, were improved by new closure devices. We had new anticoagulant agents and blood thinners in conjunction with the new procedures."

Fast-forward to 2020 and interventional cardiology is even more advanced, thanks primarily to further miniaturization, as

David explains: "[In the 1990s], you would stay in the hospital for three or four days. Now, it's three to four hours. We can go through your wrist and you can stand up immediately." Just as in the 1990s, the procedures remain imaging-driven.

David notes another key change for interventional cardiologists through the years:

"Patients are doing far better with heart attacks now than when I started. We've noted that part of the heart is being deprived of oxygen during a heart attack, so the quicker you restore oxygen, the better people's outcomes are. From the time of a patient's first medical contact, we are notified by phone and can see the patient's EKG from the field via an app. We all scramble—it's a fireman's mentality—so that from the time a patient hits the door to the time we open the vessel, it's no more than 45 minutes. It used to be 90 minutes."

One more thing that has changed: While David was hired as one of two interventionalists for CGoM in 1996, in 2020, there are six—and that's just at the practice's East Memphis location.

EXPANSION AND AN EASTWARD DRIFT

"In July 1979, Baptist Memorial Hospital East opened and we opened a second, small office there. I was assigned to manage that office. Moving into the 1980s, the Baptist East location turned out to be quite popular with physicians as well as patients." —Jan Turner, M.D., retired from Stern Cardiovascular Foundation

As the decade passed from the 1980s to the '90s, the expanding practice began to feel growing pains. Doctors cultivated patient relationships in larger numbers while Stern's ancillary services became more robust, requiring more space.

Pam Glover's recollections from the Stern Clinical Lab at the time provide context. The lab was working out of an office on the eighth floor of Baptist Memorial Medical Center Downtown. Stern's main clinic was located on the sixth floor. "Every hour, the main clinic was responsible for running up two flights of stairs to bring us samples. Research and Transcription were up there with us because Stern had started growing and we were out of space," Pam recalls.

When 930 Madison Avenue opened, CGoM seized the opportunity to expand closeby, albeit cautiously. As Dan Caldwell remembers, "We built a pretty large new office in the medical center next to the hospital. Baptist had built a new office building right next to us. They really wanted us in the new building, but we felt things were moving east."

Given the rapid rate at which the practice was growing, the move would prove to be a stop-gap. The Clinical Lab, for example, was given an entire floor in the new building. "We could get samples faster and turn them around faster. Patients could get results while they were here, depending on the test," Pam explains. But then the lab upgraded to a bigger analyzer, and hired a third person.

The Cardiology Group of Memphis' need for additional space coincided with Baptist's an-

nouncement that it would vacate downtown Memphis for its East campus—followed by the subsequent mass migration of medical practices and services to the city's eastern edge. As a temporary solution, CGoM moved much of its operation to the Baptist East location—80 Humphreys Center Drive—in 1996. The arrangement lasted several years, buying time for the group to plan its next move.

THE LIPID CLINIC

Around the same time, CGoM added another critical in-house offering: the Lipid Clinic. It won't surprise you to learn that Tom Stern led the charge. "Dr. Stern was a lipid expert," Steven Gubin notes, adding, "When he started the Lipid Clinic, he was way ahead of his time."

As it had previously, Tom's foresight placed the practice at the fore of patient care. Equally, it made a radical statement on the changing nature of healthcare in the U.S. "The system doesn't want to be involved in prevention," asserts Elissa Fine, Lipid Clinic Coordinator for Stern Cardiovascular Foundation. Nevertheless, she adds, "Our group wanted to do it anyway. We carried the Lipid Clinic because it was the right thing to do."

Elissa classifies that conviction as classic Tom Stern. "He had a large view about everything," she says. At the center of that view was one core belief: Heart disease—artery disease, especially—is preventable, if we do the right things.

At the same time, Elissa remembers, Tom had his own ideas for the operation of the clinic. "But he really left it to me," she admits, referring to the clinic function and functions that she would soon be the architect of.

The role was a precise match for Elissa. After working in exercise and physiology, she felt that her calling was to combine the disciplines of exercise, nutrition and stress management. When she decided to pursue graduate studies to this end, "Memphis State popped up," Elissa remembers. Then, "a very kind person in town mentioned me to Dr. Stern. I wanted to do this and he wanted to do this and, I guess, kismet," she says.

After joining the practice, Elissa and others visited a San Diego, California, practice to study its Lipid Clinic. Upon returning to Memphis, they got to work. Elissa began setting up classes and seeing patients, but "Dr. Stern also saw everyone I saw," she remembers, underscoring Tom's commitment to his patients and the developing clinic. "As you work beside someone you understand how their brain works and understand even more how committed they are," she says of her experience working closely with the clinic's patriarch.

The establishment of CGoM's Lipid Clinic in 1993 coincided with a sea change in doctor-patient relationships. "There was an era when doctors told a patient what to do and patients often did not, or were not allowed to, ask questions. Patients weren't involved in their own care," Elissa recalls. Within CGoM, the dynamic was different, and the Lipid Clinic was emblematic of that difference. The difference hinged on a simple idea, but one that patients at the time rarely heard: "Patients have more control over this than we

do," Elissa explains, referring to lifestyle changes a majority of patients can make if they're equipped with good information. That's where the Lipid Clinic comes in: to empower patients and foster a collaborative provider-patient relationship. "We spend a lot of time helping patients understand what's going on so they will do the things it takes to prevent them. Together, this is preventable," Elissa explains.

Today, anyone—not only existing patients— can come to the Lipid Clinic. A visit usually begins with a call from Elissa to elicit health history and risk factors, discuss medications and their safety and overview basic information. Elissa might explain what a heart attack actually is, what diagnostic tests can and can't reveal . . . "all the things we do and why we're doing them," she explains. Then the in-person visits begin. To start, "we're in a group, so it's a relaxed atmosphere," Elissa explains. She gives each patient a set of their own numbers and explains what they mean. She sets exercises for each patient in the very first class. As the series of three classes unfolds, she covers the physiology of dieting, exercise and nutrition.

For Lipid Clinic patients, Elissa defines dieting as "diets that work and why." Education in this area is a process of addressing the notions patients come to class with: labeling fat as an enemy, counting calories and limiting carbohydrates, among other fads that have been absorbed through our collective consciousness. Such fads that influence patients are "a generational thing to a certain extent," Elissa explains, but there are constants she emphasizes with all of her groups: the interplay between

heart disease and other diseases, how major diseases are linked to nutrition and exercise and how food can be your friend—an update on Neuton Stern's 1950s-era advice, if you will.

The Device Clinic

While CGoM's Lipid Clinic worked with patients on the level of prevention, another of the era's new initiatives made a foray into treatment: the Device Clinic.

Dan Caldwell explains how the clinic took shape:

Originally, CGoM decided to outsource the functions of a device clinic. In time, Dan recaps, "We felt like it was better to bring [that function] into our office for better interrogation. We bought software and some pacer equipment and outfitted an office, and that was the establishment of our formal pacer clinic."

Pamela Burks, now Director of Nursing for Stern Cardiovascular Foundation, joined the practice in 1993. "We had one person interrogating then," she recalls. Which begs the question: How did a one-person clinic grow into the team of seven doctors, seven nurses and three support personnel who power Stern's Device Clinic today?

"It's constantly evolving," Pamela explains, adding, "Our doctors are on the cutting edge. Our EP doctors are heavily involved with Dr. Frank McGrew to bring new studies to help our patients. All of our EPs attend Heart Rhythm Society meetings where they go brainstorm with other physicians around the world around new technology and bring it back to see if Stern would like to take that initiative. As busy as they are taking care of their patients, our doctors find time to stay up on current treatment modalities, new technology, FDA approval . . . and if it's something they believe in, they really get behind it through research."

(For laymen, EP is short for electrophysiologist, a doctor who implants pacemakers, defibrillators and implantable loops.)

Pamela cites one example of the connection between Stern's research arm and its EP doctors: "CRT [cardiac resynchronization therapy] devices started as a house trial within Stern. Now it's very common, and understood that patients with congestive heart failure may benefit from adding leads to help improve the pumping function of the heart," she explains.

"I see physicians going down the hall to talk to our EP doctors—it's very collaborative at Stern." — Pamela Burks

From her experience as an EP nurse to her current post overseeing Stern's Device Clinic, Pamela has observed—from the frontline—advancements in technology as well as in physician skill. When CRT implantation was new, she reports, "Every heart is different, so we would have to block off a schedule for four hours, and there are only eight hours in a day. Now, our EP doctors may do three or four CRTs in one day. They're very skilled with so many different types of hearts."

In 2003, Stern Cardiovascular nurse Regina Owen contributed an article to EP Lab Digest chronicling the growth of Stern's Device Clinic. From the article:

"For the year 2000, Stern Cardiovascular Center recorded 375 ICD [implantable cardioverter defibrillator] patient follow-up checks. As a result of broadened indications for defibrillator implants, the number of follow-up checks grew to 942 in 2001, and then to 1,305 in 2002. We are projected to exceed 1,645 by the end of 2003, a more than 430% increase over a period of three years. During the same period, pacemaker follow-up visits have grown by 32%."

In the article, Regina also proudly shared Stern's success implementing Medtronic's CareLink Network. The web-based initiative enabled remote monitoring for patients and streamlined patient management for Stern's growing practice.

How does Regina's snapshot compare to the clinic's current output?

Today, there are more than 10,000 Stern Device Clinic patients

They're seen across nine locations, including:

Three free-standing clinics: Stern's main Wolf River location and two DeSoto County, Mississippi, locations

Six additional locations serviced by device reps who travel to outlying clinics in order to interrogate patients' devices

The day-to-day business is a flurry of device reps reporting back, or nurses forming reports based on the reps' interrogations, checking existing patients per the protocol and on-boarding new patients. Home monitoring is an entrenched and critical piece. As Pamela explains:

"The patient leaves the hospital with the home monitor, or it's mailed to them. In two weeks, they come to our office to make sure they're healing, but most importantly, we interrogate the device, checking the settings and seeing if the patient has any arrhythmias. The next time, the patient reports from home and our nurses retrieve the report from the web."

It's a true team effort, bringing together the patient and his or her Device Clinic nurse, EP doctor and cardiologist.

Yet, for all of the technology it has helped to advance, Stern's Device Clinic has maintained its growth by keeping a personal touch with patients. As Pamela reflects:

"Stern has hired RNs for the Device Clinic for their critical thinking skills. They can review medications and implants. But sometimes patients come in and [need] a nurse to take it to ground zero for them, explaining, 'The reason you got this device is . . .' We encourage patients to bring family members and we really try to make the patient understand and be a participant in their own care with the device. They have a number they can call and either a secretary or nurse will respond. Patients get attached to our Device Clinic nurses because they are so caring."

LEADING ON THE LEADING EDGE

"When Tom Stern was in his 80s and I was a resident, I would round with him. He was always up to date with the latest things. McGrew does just like Tom Stern did—he stays current. He goes to meetings. He's still relevant in research. These older guys, they have a young heart, an enthusiasm for their profession and for life. That's the legacy: Stern is always at the forefront." —James Klemis, M.D., Stern Cardiovascular Foundation

As Tom Stern's medical assistant and nurse of 32 years, Randy Meeks saw firsthand how so much innovation within the practice originated with him. "He wanted the echo, the Holter machine, nuclear medicine, the pacer clinic, 'George' [the first office computer], the lab the way we have it—Dr. Stern was the one who thought we should embrace innovation," Randy remembers.

Steven Gubin echoes Randy: "Tom Stern was always ahead of the curve, looking at things that no one else was thinking about at the time. When he was in his 70s, we were talking about getting into CTA of the coronary arteries. Before we did it, we wanted to go over to Little Rock. Usually, it's the young guys doing this, so I asked Dr. Stern, 'Do you want to go over? This would be great for the group.' He went with me to look at it."

Yet, as previously noted, Tom Stern wasn't motivated by the prospect of being first-to-market for the sake of being first. Randy interpreted Tom's motivation as a direct inheritance from his father, Neuton Stern. As when Neuton introduced the first echocardiogram to Memphis—a symbol for the advancement of cardiology—Tom advocated for developments he believed would advance the specialty. At the same time, Tom championed initiatives he believed would be critical to the future of his own group: "He was for everything being full-service,"

Randy says, adding, "It was partly a quality-control [issue]: If we do it in-house, we know it's done right. But it was also being able to offer services you should be able to if you're a premier provider." James Klemis agrees with Randy's take. "To build this practice, the older guys laid a good foundation: The patient is first. It's not about ego or saying, 'Look what we have.' What we do and offer is so our patients don't have to go to Cleveland Clinic or Mayo; it's so they can come right here," James asserts.

In 1992, The Commercial Appeal asked 2,247 Shelby County physicians "whom they would turn to for medical care. The survey listed 17 medical specialties and four primary care areas. [Thomas Stern] was the physician named most often by colleagues asked [whom] they would turn to for treatment of heart disease." Jan Turner, David Holloway and Frank McGrew also ranked in the survey's top six, each receiving a minimum of 10 votes.

The advancement of technology. The progression of cardiology. The development of the practice. There was, of course, one driving factor behind them all. "In thinking ahead, Dr. Stern just wanted the best for the patient. He always put the patient first," Steven Gubin says.

In the realm of research, Frank McGrew never shied from taking the lead. "I appreciate Frank McGrew. He's one of the original guys but he keeps doing the research. He was a big mentor . . . always enthusiastic about what we were doing," James says, remembering how McGrew supported his involvement in national trials related to James' specialty, carotid

stenting: "He would send me patients. This really encouraged me. He could have been threatened by youth. But he enjoyed helping the young guys up the mountain rather than playing king of the mountain."

The big picture, 100 years in, looks like this, as described by Steven Gubin:

"We have the best of both worlds. We have an academic environment in which we participate in numerous research protocols, allowing our patients access to advanced cardiac care before these therapies are available to the general public. Most of our cardiologists sub-specialize so that we staff experts in different areas of cardiology. I think that's something that sets us apart from other groups. And we offer services that make it easier for patients to access cardiology care—multiple clinics, the dispensary, outreach."

. . . which sounds much like Tom Stern's version, one reason that in 1997, the Cardiology Group of Memphis changed its name to the Stern Cardiovascular Center.

This would be a nice place to insert the list of presidents that Dr. Gubin would like to see in the manuscript. Stern will need to construct this on their end.

CLINICAL COLLABORATION

In 1998, Stern Cardiovascular Center partnered with Sutherland Cardiology Clinic and St. Francis' Cardiology Associates to staff an outpatient cath lab facility. The idea for the facility originated with Stern Executive Director Fred Klyman. As Melissa Reaves, now CFO of Stern Cardiovascular Foundation, remembers:

"Dr. Klyman was adamant about having a joint venture between us, Sutherland and Cardiology Associates. To have a cath lab, you have to have a certificate of need (CON, a legal document required before an acquisition, expansion or creation of a new facility can occur). Baptist and Methodist already had cath labs, but St. Francis was willing to have this outpatient diagnostic facility on their campus."

Inside the facility, the groups alternated days to conduct all of their catheterization procedures. Melissa explains, "We had two days, Sutherland had two days and Cardiology Associates had one day; we had a whole structure with expenses coordinated out."

For all of the finely tuned logistics, Melissa describes how the physicians granted each other leeway for the good of their patients. "If we had an opening in a day and a Sutherland or Cardiology Associates physician had to have a patient in, we would say 'go ahead' and they would do the same."

After a decade of successful collaboration, Sutherland began working toward its forthcoming venture with Methodist Le Bonheur Healthcare; Stern and Baptist would soon hold similar conversations. Yet, the period stands as a shining example of intergroup cooperation in Memphis. "For competing cardiologists, it worked very, very well," Melissa affirms.

DR. FRED KLYMAN

At a glance, Fred Klyman may not have been an obvious choice to help manage a cardiology practice. With a doctorate in education, Fred served as a professor and even developed an innovative curriculum for the Memphis Police Department Training Academy. Yet as his career evolved, he gained experience in healthcare, working on contracts between hospitals, doctors and insurers.

It was this experience that called Fred to mind when Marty Grusin was searching for a partner in his work with Stern. "I told Fred: 'You can help both sides—getting doctors organized but also working with the insurers who pay them—and I'll handle the legal aspects until you get a feel.' We worked together jointly for a year, first figuring out the challenges and then the solutions," Marty recalls.

From the cath lab you read about in this chapter to the new building and rebranding you'll read about in the next, Fred's solutions were rooted in a clear vision for Stern Cardiovascular Center. And while high-profile projects demonstrated the outcomes, Fred's solutions always started with the fundamentals. As Debbie Eddlestone remembers, "When Dr. Klyman arrived in late 1996, he pulled everything together by creating a board of directors and administrators, a mix of insiders and outsiders, that would answer to him." With the foundation shored up, Fred was able to move forward with physical solutions. In addition to the cath lab, Fred secured land in Germantown and began building at DeSoto and Wolf River. "He had a vision that Germantown would be Memphis' medical corridor. He entrenched our group in a new community that eventually became the medical corridor he envisioned," Debbie says.

For his foresight, Debbie calls Fred Klyman a visionary and a cowboy. She also calls him her mentor, and a pivotal player in Stern's rebirth. "He gave me the open books and allowed me to flourish. When our foundation almost cracked, Dr. Klyman came in and stabilized it so Stern could continue on."

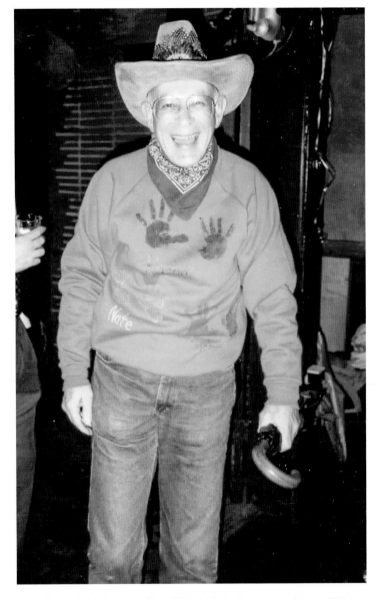

"Annual Holiday party (Dec '92 I think) -the theme was Country/Western dancing complete with an instructor. Most of us were in theme wear. Dr. Stern made a fashionably late entry wearing jeans and a cowboy hat and the crowd "went wild"! Not expected at all and many could not believe that he owned a cowboy hat (it was his) or jeans."

Photo thanks to Randy Meeks

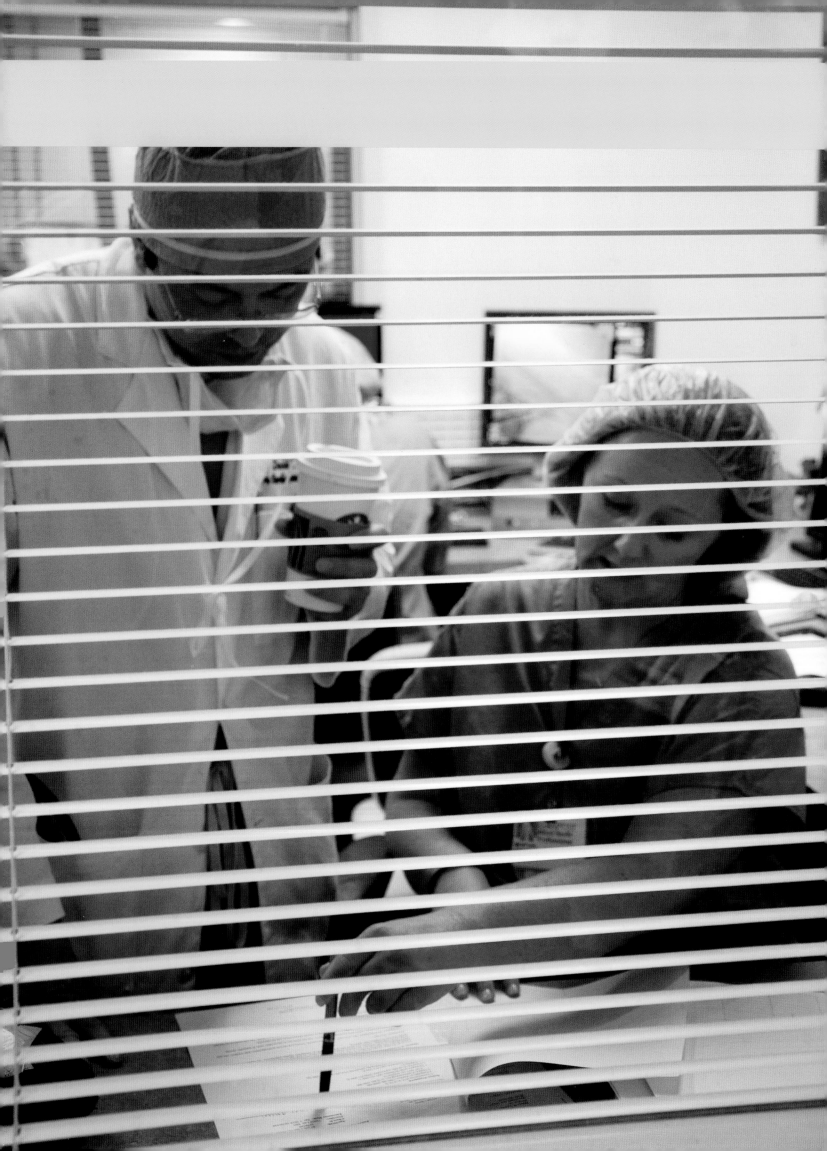

Chapter 8: The 2000s: A Practice for the New Millennium

B Y 2000, SUDDEN DEATH FROM A 'HEART ATTACK' IN AN OTHERWISE HEALTHY PERSON WAS LESS COMMON THAN IT HAD BEEN A DECADE EARLIER. NEW TECHNOLOGIES SCREENED FOR ATHEROSCLEROTIC HEART DISEASE, AND INVASIVE CARDIOLOGISTS COULD DILATE AND PLACE STENTS IN OCCLUDED CORONARY ARTERIES, CHANGING THE OUTLOOK FOR PATIENTS. AS PATIENTS LIVED LONGER WITH A BETTER QUALITY OF LIFE, THEY REQUIRED ONGOING CARE THAT INCREASED THE NEED FOR CARDIOLOGISTS." —PATRICIA LAPOINTE MCFARLAND AND MARY ELLEN PITTS, EXCERPTED FROM MEMPHIS MEDICINE: A HISTORY OF SCIENCE AND SERVICE

As the new millennium dawned, changes emerged on the horizon for Stern Cardiovascular Center—and for the entire ecosystem of healthcare in Memphis. The year 2000 marked the end of era, when Baptist Memorial Health Care officially closed its flagship location in downtown Memphis. The location where orthopedists, neurologists and cardiologists—

starting with Neuton Stern—pioneered their fields; where the first attached physician's building, the first automatic elevator and the first computer for account billing debuted among our country's hospitals; where Lisa Marie Presley was born and Elvis Presley was pronounced dead. The building would be imploded in 2005. But its beginnings in 1912 barely

pre-date the dawn of Neuton Stern's practice downtown. With the move of Baptist, Stern fully vacated downtown Memphis in July 2000, adopting as its new headquarters the office at 80 Humphreys Center Drive.

Yet, some things remained unchanged as ever, and those things tended to distinguish Stern among other cardiovascular practices

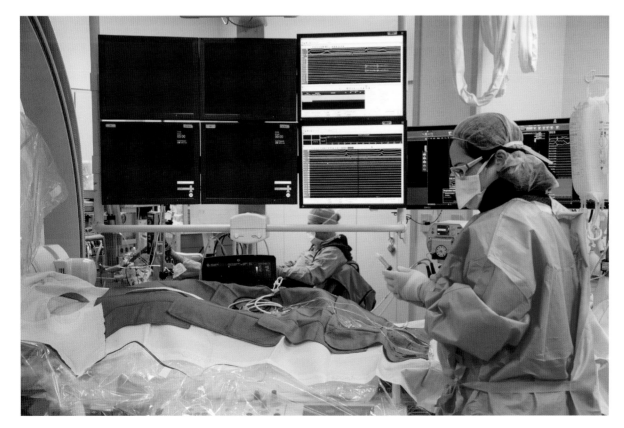

◀ Scenes from the operating room at Batpist Hospital

Photos by Stephanie Norwood

of the time. "In the early 2000s, every cardiologist did everything, but not here. We thought you could do better to focus on one area," Steven Gubin explains. That philosophy guided Stern's recruiting efforts through the decade as the practice responded to the increased need for cardiologists noted by authors McFarland and Pitts. That, and a nationwide scope: "We had university connections all over the country," Steven offers, adding, "Not all of our talent was homegrown."

A New "Class" of Cardiologists

In 2003, the first of those out-of-home recruits was Arie Szatkowski, M.D. As he recalls:

"[While] training during my fellowship at Columbia Presbyterian in New York City, I put my CV on the American College of Cardiology website and started getting phone calls from Steven Gubin. I had absolutely no intention of going to Memphis and no plans whatsoever to leave New York City. I had this perception of everything in the South being backwards, [like] we'd be practicing in a barn. But Gubin called me probably every single day. I thought, 'I'll go for a weekend, hang out on Beale Street, see Graceland and it'll be on their dime.' I visited and had a really wonderful experience. The weekend that I came in, Steven set up a dinner with Mayor Willie Herenton and the Lieutenant Governor of Tennessee. There I was having dinner thinking, 'Mayor Giuliani would never do this!'"

Arie remembers being "totally impressed" by the history of the practice. "That got my mind thinking about things outside of New York," he admits, though he took the Stern job with no intention of staying in Memphis for an extended time. Perhaps because of (or in spite of) that, he set into motion a chain reaction in recruiting that built the next generation of Stern physicians.

Arie remembers how one of those early recruits came to be: "Walking through the halls at Baptist, I walked into this old-school clinician talking about his cousin at Columbia. I asked, 'Which attending is that?' and he said, 'Dan Otten.'" As it turns out, Dan had trained a year below Arie, and Arie had recruited Dan to the fellowship at Columbia. Arie then helped bring Dan to Stern, his second recruit following Jason Infeld, M.D. Shortly after came Drs. James Klemis, Holger Salazar and Jennifer Morrow. "As we developed this pipeline to young folks, the group started to grow," Arie says. Yet, Arie draws a direct line from Neuton and Tom Stern to the group's 21st century recruits: Like Stern's legacy doctors, who were "always on the forefront of medicine," in Arie's words, the new recruits were "fresh minds looking at medicine from a more modern slant," he explains. Whether a physician represented the old or new guard, they could find common ground: "That's one thing about Stern: You never sit back and ride on what's happening," Arie shares.

James Klemis shared his decision to come on board. After completing medical school in Augusta, the Georgia native "wanted a change of pace and came on a lark" to Memphis, where he trained with Tom Stern, followed by additional training in New York City. James paints the contrast between the two cities as stark: "In New York City, it was all about them. Tom Stern was equally accomplished, but he genuinely took the time to teach us. He really cared." After training, James launched a nationwide search for his future practice. He describes what he found upon returning to Stern: "This world-class group attracted people from all the top schools. I knew how hard they worked, but there was equal opportunity, unlike the model where the old guys dominate and the young guys work a lot." Arie attributes the cultivation of this atmosphere to Steven Gubin.

James remembers having one more criterion throughout his search: "I wanted a mixture of private practice, but also big-level research like you get at an academic center," he says. He found that in a mentoring relationship with Frank McGrew. "The combination of all of these things and the ability to practice like I wanted to," James recalls, decided him. He joined Stern in 2006 as an interventional cardiologist.

"There's a quote in science that says: People are where they are because of the people who mentored them. I had the training, but without Stern, I was just another guy. I was new. I needed the support of the group to get the word out about what I could do. After me came more doctors who could do new things. I was a cog in the wheel moving things forward, and now several more have come who push the group forward. The group supports us as we work together." —James Klemis, M.D.

The timing was opportune, considering Stern's tradition of walking the leading edge and James' focus: "In cardiology, every five or 10 years, there are new breakthroughs," he explains, continuing, "In the early- to mid-2000s, carotid stenting was the breakthrough. I was the first at Stern to do carotid stenting; the first to do atrial septal defect and PFO closure. My expertise expanded the practice and kept us at the forefront," James says.

In many ways, the decade's new class of recruits represented a bridging of the old and new guard. Jennifer Morrow, who joined in 2006, explains:

"Jan Turner was one of my best friends' dads. That was my knowledge of Stern growing up: It was our parents' generation. I'm from Memphis but did my training elsewhere and moved away for a long time. I didn't join Stern right away but very quickly realized I should have: Jan Turner talked to me a lot and encouraged me to come. I was at the forefront of the new generation, but it was an interesting perspective that we got to work with the older guys, too. We could share new technology as the young guys and then turn around to Dr. Holloway and ask, 'Have you seen one of these in your career?' He'd remember the name of the patient, what happened and how they were diagnosed."

A Patient's Perspective: Mark Agostinelli

When Mark Agostinelli—fresh off of his first year of college—presented with high blood pressure, his hometown doctor recognized that Mark's condition was one he couldn't diagnose. That

doctor, practicing in Clarksdale, Mississippi, referred Mark to Tom Stern. Mark remembers their initial meeting around 1983:

"Dr. Stern heard a heart murmur. He checked my blood pressure in my legs and my blood pressure in my arms and it was different. I don't know how he knew to check that but he knew that I had a closing of the aortic artery. I was 18 years old."

Mark underwent surgery as a result of the diagnosis and began seeing Tom Stern regularly. The visits required precious time away from Mark's livelihood of farming cotton and beans, driving from Clarksdale to Memphis. His wife, Leigh Ann, accompanied him to every appointment.

"We would sit in the waiting room and people would look at us like, 'What are you doing here?' because we were the youngest patients Dr. Stern had," Leigh Ann laughs. "But he would make us feel extra special," she remembers, describing how Tom would proclaim, upon seeing the couple in the office, "Oh! My grandchildren are coming in!"

Through the years, Mark and Tom adopted other familiar patterns. One was an exercise to hone cardiologists in training. "Dr. Stern would always have students following him around," Mark remembers, explaining, "Because I had a unique heart problem, he would get them to come listen to my heart and ask them what they heard to see if they could pick up on what my troubles were." Asked if any student ever accurately diagnosed his condition, Mark remembers a few students offering possibilities, and Tom smiling slightly. "He wanted them to

listen, and he had the patience of Job," Mark says.

The pair liked to joke with each other, too. "He had his own sense of humor. He would ask me how the crop was and I would say, 'Dr. Stern, you know I'm not going to tell you it's good. You're going to charge me too much!' and he would just laugh. That was a joke between us every time we would go in," Mark recalls fondly.

Nearing 25 years together as doctor and patient, Mark liked to tease Tom about his age. "You're getting old now," Mark would joke, following up with, "Who's going to take your place?" This, too, made Tom laugh, but he took Mark's future care seriously and crafted a plan. It fell into place at just the right time, for Tom's own health would soon decline.

"When Dr. Stern got sick, I was having a very hard time working the farm. I had no energy so I called him and said, 'I need to come to the office.' He said, 'No, you're going to go to the hospital.'" Mark rebutted that he didn't have time to leave the farm for the hospital. But it rained that night and kept Mark from working. As it turns out, Tom was hospitalized at the time himself. The Agostinellis wondered whom they would see. Tom called them from his own hospital room to say, "Don't you worry about it. We're going to take care of y'all. I have the best doctor for you." It was Jennifer Morrow.

When a patient sees the same two doctors over the course of four decades, shared experiences mount. "They saved my life a couple of times," Mark says. And yet, Mark and Leigh Ann have been deeply impressed by the character—not merely by the clinical skill—of their Stern physicians. "Dr. Stern was just a fine man. He listened to you. He had a way of making you feel like everything was going to be okay. He just became part of the family," Mark shares.

Leigh Ann echoes Mark's sentiment. Receiving the news of Tom Stern's passing, she remembers, "It was like one of my family members had died." But, she adds, "Dr. Stern always said he was going to take care of us when he quit practicing." By transitioning Mark to Jennifer Morrow, Tom ensured that the cycle of care and friendship would continue. Mark, accompanied by Leigh Ann, has been seeing Jennifer now for 13 years and counting. Reminiscent of Tom's grandfatherly connection to the Agostinellis, Jennifer has taken her own family to visit Mark and Leigh Ann on their farm.

EXCELLENCE IN PATIENT CARE

"Tom Stern's medical scholarship, teaching, research and humanistic concern for his patients has prompted the Stern Cardiovascular Center to adopt as its mission statement: 'Excellence in Cardiovascular Medicine, Research and Patient Care.'" — From the Stern Cardiovascular Foundation archives

As Mark Agostinelli's case demonstrates, Stern Cardiovascular Foundation provides an uncommon level of patient care. It's nothing new, as Nancy Hardin, employed by the practice in 1954, attests. "Dr. Neuton Stern had you in mind. You were his priority," she says.

In her time with the group, CEO Debbie Eddlestone has seen this play out time and time again. As she explains: "From Dr. Stern's time on, even to today, these doctors are willing to do the full gamut. If you ask patients who come in here, 'Who's your primary care doctor?,' they say, 'Dr. Gubin. He takes care of me for everything,' or, 'I've been seeing Dr. Holloway for 40 years. It's Dr. Holloway.' And that's how people see Stern doctors. The doctors go with it—they wouldn't send one of their patients away to somebody else; they would just take care of the patient. If you spent a day with anybody here, you would be amazed at the length that everybody is willing to go for the community and for the service that they provide."

"It's not uncommon for me to walk into an exam room and have three generations of patients right there." —Frank McGrew, M.D.

For Debbie, it calls to mind practice lore: stories passed down from the days when Tom Stern's trunk would be packed with equipment, ready for him to rush to the homes of patients in need. "He would pull up and do what had to be done," Debbie affirms. In stories such as this one, it's easy to hear the echoes of Neuton Stern knocking on patients' doors as he made house calls in the early 20th century.

Debbie explains how this level of personalized care became a throughline in the practice. As she notes, it begins with the recruitment of new doctors: Recruiting physicians gage candidates' feelings about how they want to practice because, "at the end of the day, it's about the patient and the service, not just that you see X amount of patients in a day. You get patients because of what you can do, and because you're the right doctor for them, and you develop a rapport. It's about having a relationship with your patient, not just about seeing that person as the next patient," Debbie asserts.

James Klemis expands on Debbie's assertion: "You see your patients as family. That's the ethos of Stern. I think that's the legacy of the early doctors."

BUILDING FOR THE FUTURE

In 2003, the greatest physical change in the history of the practice came, when the group moved to 8060 Wolf River Boulevard in Germantown, Tennessee. The 55,000-square-foot facility officially opened on December 1. Melissa Reaves, Stern Cardiovascular Foundation CFO, recalls the decision-making process that went into selecting the site:

"Dr. Klyman was really instrumental looking around and searching for properties close to the hospital, making sure that when physicians were in-clinic, they didn't have to travel too far. If you know anything about the area, you know there's not a whole lot of land near the hospital that the hospital doesn't own. They looked at a piece of land near where Sutherland Cardiology Clinic is now, but did not like the flood [hazard]. Then they found another area, just a bit further down Wolf River Boulevard. They liked the way it was laid out because they could make it a physician corridor," Melissa explains, referring to a "physician's row" of offices in a direct line with the hospital.

While the move created physical opportunity, it also served as the impetus for a full rebranding of the practice. Again, Fred Klyman led the charge. As Melissa recounts, "It was his vision; his push to get it done," including the adoption of official colors and a new seal for the practice, designed by Dr. Klyman himself. "We got that seal patented because Dr. Klyman wanted no one else to have it," Melissa remembers.

The rebranding also enabled one very personal tribute. When the new building opened, it opened under the practice's relatively new name: The Stern Cardiovascular Center. Steven Gubin remembers: "The day that we named the group after Dr. Stern, I heard he went home to his wife and sat down to dinner and said, 'Today, the group did a really nice thing for me.' That was it! I'm so happy he got to see the building named after him before he passed away." Susan Edelman adds a footnote to Steven's story: "Dad was adamant that the practice was named after his father and not him." Randy Meeks sees it this way: "Dr. Stern doesn't just have his name on the building because he was the primary person—it's there because he built all of this. He made it grow. It is what it is because of him."

A Somber Day

Just three years later, Tom Stern was diagnosed with lung cancer. Still, Randy Meeks remembers, "He didn't retire. He came into the office as much as he could and I would take charts to him in the evening after he was staying at home. He would tell me what to tell patients. He wanted to do that."

Tom Stern passed away on September 9, 2006, at Baptist Memorial Hospital. At the memorial service, a group of family members gathered: Tom's biological and work relations, a "family" united by the man they loved and looked up to. "The office was closed and we were all there," Nancy Cummings remembers. In fact, David Holloway, Tom's colleague since 1969, delivered a eulogy. Cindy White, Director of EHR Informatics for Stern Cardiovascular Foundation, remembers it vividly: "In front of a packed room at Temple Israel, Dr. Holloway stood up without any piece of paper and just spoke from the heart about his friend."

Jennifer Morrow had been practicing at Stern for a few years by this time. "It was an amazing thing to work with the reigning patriarch of cardiology in this city and the namesake of the clinic," she says, looking back at her earliest days in the group and the opportunity to practice alongside Tom Stern. After his death, something unexpected happened: Jennifer inherited his office. She considers it a link to him. "In my exam room, there's still his antique exam table and it's full of good stuff: His papers and diplomas are still in there because I don't want to take anything out. I think it has very good karma," she says.

The first decade of the 21st century was defined by change for Stern Cardiovascular. In addition to welcoming the next generation of cardiologists and moving into a new home, the group would add major components to its offering: an anticoagulation clinic, electronic medical records and a dispensary.

The Anticoagulation Clinic

Stern continued to blaze a pioneering trail right into the 21st century. The group's first bold move was to open one of the first Anticoagulation Clinics in Memphis. Rebecca Fleshman, one of two Stern Cardiovascular Foundation Directors of Nursing, now oversees the clinic. She began working with the group one month after Tom Stern's passing. Though she didn't have the chance to work alongside him, Rebecca understands that Tom's influence is imprinted on the work the clinic performs every day. "Stern has always been about serving the community. That was Dr. Stern's idea. The intent was for patients to have that 'this-is-your-family'-type feeling," she explains. Adding the Anticoagulation Clinic furthered that feeling by helping to build Stern's profile as a one-stop shop for patients.

In the 20 years since its creation, Stern's Anticoagulation Clinic has grown exponentially, even as some patients transition from coumadin to anticoagulants that don't require blood monitoring. Today, the clinic sees more than 5,000 patients annually. That averages out to approximately 550 patients weekly, seen by a dedicated team of six employees across three Stern locations: Wolf River, Walnut Grove and Southaven. What has driven the increase in volume of patients seen? Rebecca reports that doctors are identifying patients earlier on, but advancements in technology and the collaboration with Baptist have contributed as well.

The major advancement Rebecca refers to, of course, is home

monitoring. Of the clinic's current caseload, she explains, "We have home-monitoring patients we manage as well as patients that come into the clinic itself. That subset of patients—the ones put on home monitors or who live in rural areas and send their results in—has only grown." Following home-monitoring protocol, patients can have their tests performed in a location convenient to their homes. Stern's Anticoagulation Clinic receives the results and communicates resultant actions just as it would for in-office patients; the only difference is that those actions are communicated by phone, saving the patient the drive.

The Baptist collaboration, on the other hand, serves as a pipeline. Take the example of a new heart patient who's been seen at a Baptist location by a Stern physician. "When that patient gets out of the hospital, they automatically know to come and be seen at our clinic—even before their office visit with their primary care physician," explains Rebecca.

Despite its growing caseload, Stern's Anticoagulation Clinic has made time to reach for the highest standards. In 2016, after a battery of tests and process improvements, the team was named an Anticoagulation Center of Excellence by the Anticoagulation Forum.

Rebecca is similarly proud of the role the clinic plays in making connections and problem-solving for patients. It's an obvious benefit that Stern patients can receive so many related services under one roof. If a coumadin patient's fingerstick sample comes back at a certain level, Anticoagulation

Clinic staff can send that patient to Stern's on-site lab. Alternately, patients who need lab work can have their INR checked as part of their lab order, rather than making a separate visit to Stern's Anticoagulation Clinic. The greatest synergy of all is the clinic's ability to facilitate on-the-spot patient care. A patient visiting the Anticoagulation Clinic might say, "'I don't feel well. Can you take my blood pressure?' We'll contact the physician and nurse and say, 'This patient might need to be worked in to see you today.' There's a lot of interdepartmental work being done here," Rebecca explains.

Rebecca sees this work between Stern's internal teams, and its positive outcomes for patients, as part of the practice's century-old credo: "Doing the right thing and keeping the community connection alive: That, to me, is what's kept us going for 100 years," she shares.

ELECTRONIC HEALTH RECORDS

The history of electronic health records in the U.S. dates to the mid-1960s, when Lockheed developed what was known as a clinical information system. The history of EHR at Stern, unsurprisingly, starts with Tom Stern.

"When I started [at Stern] in 1992, Dr. Stern was already looking at EMRs," recalls Cindy White, Director of EHR Informatics for Stern Cardiovascular. White admits that, at the time, she was unfamiliar with the concept. She'd been hired as a medical transcriptionist, and in the early 1990s, the state of medical record-keeping was decidedly analog. As Cindy recollects:

"Back then, dictation was on a microcassette. Doctors would use the dictaphone and send us a set of paper charts with the cassette tape on top. The transcription would be printed on both sides of the paper to save room in the chart. We had a ruler to measure where the transcription should start on the last piece of paper in the chart. The transcriptionist would then space down in WordPerfect 5.0 and feed this last page through our HP deskjets."

Then in 1998, Stern acquired a new Manager for Medical Records and Transcription, Lisa Ciaramitaro. Her first order of business was moving the practice to a new system: digital telephone dictation. Stern physicians were already using a similar system at the hospital; developing an internal system was a matter of mimicking functions that doctors had already begun to feel familiar with. Under the new system, a doctor would call in, enter an identification number and dictate over the phone. Gone were the tapes, though Cindy remembers having to confiscate more than one dictaphone following the change. The dictations were stored on servers and an interface server transferred the records to Allscripts. Inside Stern, those stacks of paper charts topped with cassettes also became obsolete as the team introduced dividers and prongs for better organized charts.

The transition to digital telephone dictation was a precursor to the group's shift to electronic health records. The shift began in 2002, and transcription was one of the first functions the practice would on-board. "It was a journey," Cindy says, describing general and technical trials early on: "There were long hours trying to get everything caught up with the conversion. There were issues with formatting: The transcription could look one way in the record, but print differently. It would drive Dr. Stern crazy." Cindy remembers when the long hours and troubleshooting began to pay off: "I can remember standing upstairs and Dr. Stern called me from across the hall. He walked up to me, gave me a hug and said, 'I really appreciate how hard you've been working on this project.' That was so kind, I'll never forget it."

When Debbie Eddlestone was named Inside Memphis Business CEO of the Year in 2017, the tribute cited her work to remake the business operation of Stern Cardiovascular Foundation, starting with the digitization of medical records. Reflecting back to that period, Debbie says the keys were being inclusive: recognizing that every single person at Stern, not just the clinical staff of doctors and nurses, plays a part in supporting the shift to EHR.

Part of the transition was scanning and indexing every existing paper chart—one by one. The group's new facility had been designed to include a spacious file room, but the need for such a room was quickly evaporating. Within a few years, the transition team cleared the entire room of every physical file and Stern's business office moved into the space. Susan Edelman's children (Tom Stern's grandchildren) were enlisted in the effort, scanning old files as a summer job.

Moving the lab onto Stern's inchoate EHR system came next. As Stern on-boarded more

functions within the practice, the functionality of EHR expanded. Cindy trained as a super-user to put those new functions, and then some, to work for Stern. She now custom-develops modules to fit the unique needs of users within the practice. Consider this example she shared:

"We developed a note for our Anticoagulation Clinic that adjusts a patient's dosage based on their finger stick. When our Anticoagulation Clinic enters those results, it creates a flowsheet of the INR results in the patient's chart. There's a company that has a module for this, but Rebecca couldn't get them to do what our note does today."

Integrating practice functions remains a priority for Cindy's Informatics Team. Registration. Scheduling. Lab orders and results. Pacemaker and implantable cardiac monitor (ICM) reports for the Device Clinic. Leading into Stern's centennial year, all of these functions have been successfully integrated, and Cindy's team is actively pursuing additional opportunities. At the time of her interview for this book, she was finishing an integration of event and Holter monitor readings. "We're slowly reducing the amount of paper we scan and index," she reports.

While Informatics pushes Stern into the future of practice management and environmental consciousness, its full embrace of EHR—with myriad implications for better serving and caring for patients—gives an unmistakable nod to Stern's timeless practice of putting patients first.

What does medical transcription look like in Stern's centennial year? According to Cindy:

"Most of the doctors who still dictate use an app on their phones. There's even an app that allows doctors to use their phones as microphones and sync to their computers. If they're logged into the EMR, they can do their dictation right there. For new providers, we help them create templates, text macros—all kinds of shortcuts that help them with their documentation. They'll dictate, but now we have sections in our notes so they'll use text templates, and discrete data auto-pulls into the record so they don't have to dictate that anymore."

As Stern's Director of Quality and Compliance, Colleen LaCroix is in constant interaction with the EHR and Cindy's team. She came to work for the practice in 2004. Reflecting back over the years, Colleen says, "It's amazing to see how we've grown from charts on a rack in a wall to this electronic environment that helps us better manage and care for our patients."

Expanding Roles for Nurse Practitioners

Raquel Vaughan, a Family Nurse Practitioner and board-certified Acute Care Nurse Practitioner, first joined Stern in 2003. At the time, the practice's nurse practitioners were primarily hospital-based. Raquel's goal was to provide clinic-based care, and she eventually moved on to pursue it.

In her time away, two things happened: Raquel missed her work at Stern, and Steven Gubin invited her to come back, working strictly in-clinic. Raquel's return in January 2005 signaled the practice's shift toward utilizing nurse practitioners in-hospital as well as in-clinic. It further signaled the beginning of a robust nurse practitioner program inside the practice. Raquel remembers that, shortly after her return, "Other physicians started saying, 'I think I could utilize a nurse practitioner in my practice, not just at the hospital.' There were 14 physicians and eight to 10 nurse practitioners at the time at Stern. Today, there are close to 50. We now allow nurse practitioners to be hospital-based or clinic-based, and a few do both," she explains.

As Raquel has observed and experienced, the benefits of a program so robust are numerous. Seeing patients routinely in-clinic allows Stern's nurse practitioners to build meaningful relationships with patients, the aspect of practice that Raquel deems the most rewarding. At intervals, nurse practitioners collaborate on advanced initiatives with physicians. (During her collaboration with Steven Gubin, physician and nurse practitioner worked together on a prevention initiative, offering advanced testing to identify and improve outcomes for high-risk patients.) The sum of these interactions allows the nurse practitioners to play a critical role in patients' continuity of care. Raquel says it works because, "Stern physicians and nurse practitioners have a great mutual respect for one another. It takes all of us to be able to give that quality of care that Stern wants to deliver."

The Dispensary

Debbie Eddlestone explains how Stern's decision to add a dispensary came about. "In a meeting one night, we were talking about one of the biggest problems doctors were seeing: noncompliance in patients with their medications," Eddlestone remembers. When the group examined the factors behind that noncompliance, they noticed the number of patients who were receiving transportation to their appointments at Stern. "If you get transportation here, the transportation may pick you up at 5 or 6 o'clock at night. They're not going to take you to Walgreens to get your prescription filled," Debbie explains. At the same time, restrictions on pharmaceutical companies diminished the number of samples they were able to pass along to Stern, and thus, to Stern patients. The net effect? "Patients weren't starting on their medications, and we couldn't have enough samples here for the amount of people we see," Debbie notes, remembering the group's next steps. The key was looking to Allscripts. The healthcare IT giant had, of late, facilitated Stern's early adoption of electronic medical records, but Allscripts got its start as a medication packaging company. An envoy of Stern employees toured the facility. Upon discovering Allscripts' on-site dispensary, Debbie remembers a consensus among her cohorts: "That was very interesting to us, for the future of Stern," she says.

The discovery led to the creation of Stern's own on-site dispensary in 2007. For laypersons who might think of it as a pharmacy, Debbie clarifies: "We don't have to have a pharmacist. We only do pre-packaged cardiac medication. You're not going to come here and get antibiotics or anything like that. But it means the world to somebody who's got transportation that's not going to pick them up until the evening . . . at least they were able to get to the dispensary and get their medication." With the addition, the practice moved closer to realizing Tom Stern's blueprint of a full-service clinic. "It wasn't because we wanted to be a pharmacy," Debbie asserts, adding, "It really started as a convenience to the patient."

Today, Stern Cardiovascular Foundation's Dispensary is staffed by five employees, including Director Lindsey Williams, two pharmacy technicians and two nurses. One of those nurses is Tom Stern's former transcriptionist, Nancy Cummings. Echoing Debbie, Nancy describes the benefit of the Stern Dispensary: "It's an advantage for our patients, especially if it's [a medication] the doctor wants to get started today. On their way home, they just stop by the dispensary and pick it up. We run it on their insurance just like any other pharmacy," she explains. Nancy describes unexpected benefits for Stern patients, too: Whether it's apprising patients of coupons offered by drug companies or demonstrating a personal investment in patients' lives, "we get attached," Nancy says, recalling times the Dispensary staff has called spouses to check on patients, sent cards and even attended funeral visitations—calling to mind the Stern way of treating patients like family.

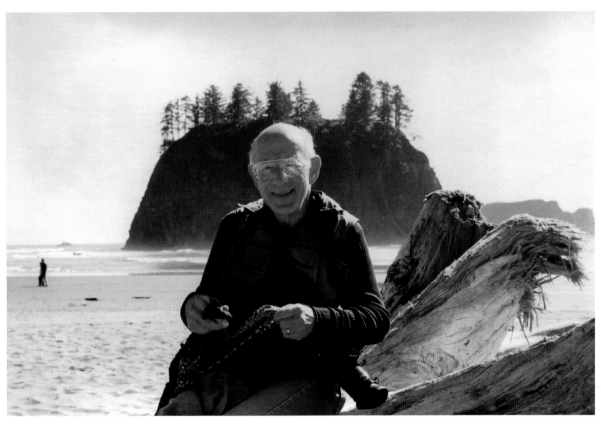

▲ Tom Stern
Photo thanks to David Stern

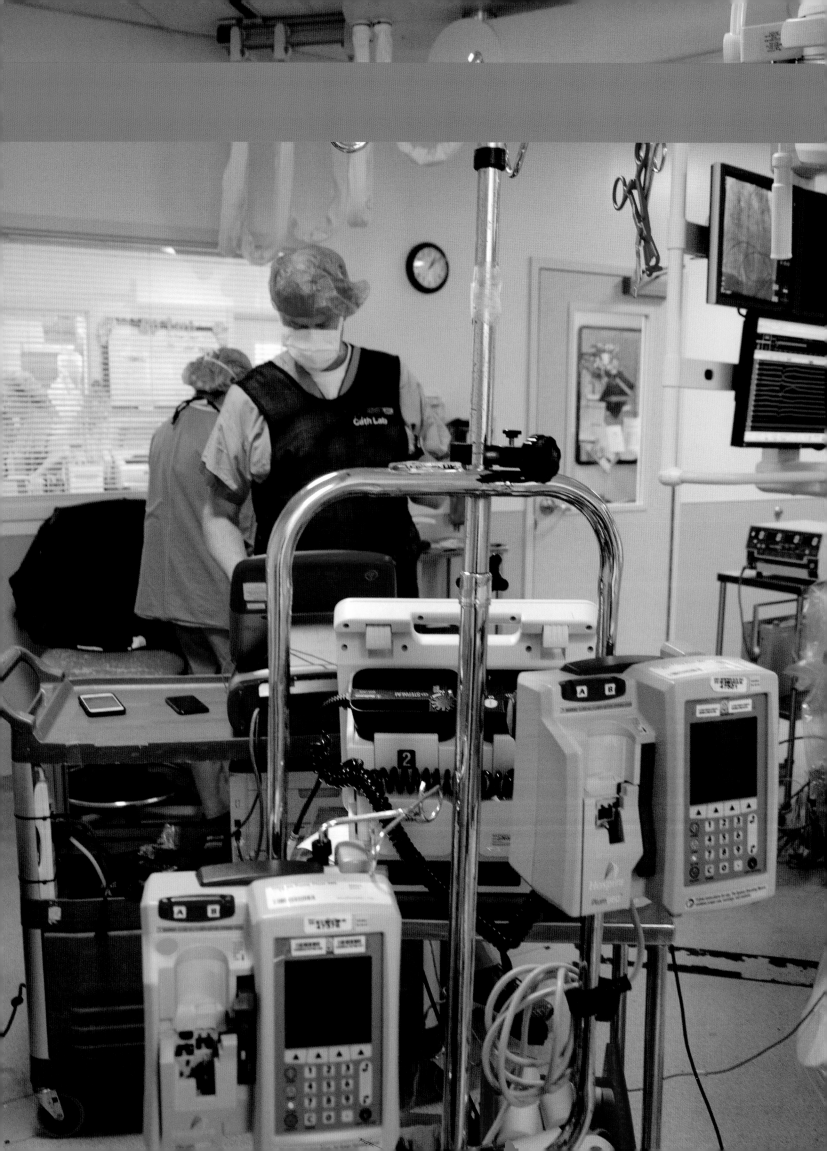

L EADERSHIP IN CARDIOLOGY HAS ALSO BEEN A LONGSTANDING TRADITION SINCE THE EARLY DAYS OF BAPTIST MEMORIAL HOSPITAL. WHILE PRACTICING AT BAPTIST IN THE EARLY 1900s, DR. NEUTON STERN FOUNDED THE CARDIOLOGY PRACTICE THAT HAS SINCE BECOME THE WELL-KNOWN STERN CARDIOVASCULAR CENTER." —PATRICIA LaPOINTE McFARLAND AND MARY ELLEN PITTS, EXCERPTED FROM MEMPHIS MEDICINE: A HISTORY OF SCIENCE AND SERVICE

Leading into 2010, it wasn't just the practice of cardiology that was changing. "Medicine was transforming," Arie Szatkowski remembers. "You wish you could just be a doctor, but you can't do that unless you find a way to maintain your autonomy while delivering your best care," he adds. In response, Arie and Jason Infeld set to work. "We saw the obstacles that would keep the practice from flourishing and moving forward. We looked at how we handled our

finances and quality; asked if our docs were following the standard of care . . . things that were mattering more and more. We presented to the senior partners, [saying], 'Here's the state of what's happening and here's where we have to be if we want to survive,'" Arie says. It wasn't easy, but incrementally, the proposal was adopted.

Pillars of the proposal were informed by several sources, including attendance at national meetings for private groups with

outpatient cardiac catheterization labs. As Arie reports:

"We knew we wouldn't be able to sustain our lab with private cuts. Those meetings are where we began to learn about other opportunities and ways we could survive. Small cardiology groups would talk about healthcare law, cardiology care in terms of payments, patient choice, consumerism, technology . . . all the things that are evolving so rapidly in our world. From these meetings, we

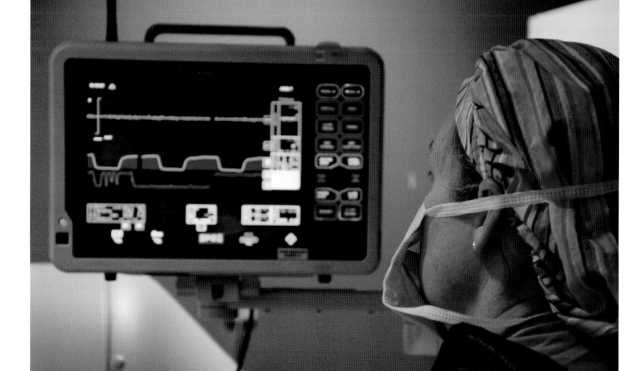

◀ Scenes from the operating room at Batpist Hospital

Photos by Stephanie Norwood

would come back with a world of knowledge."

COLLABORATION WITH BAPTIST MEMORIAL HEALTH CARE

One idea sparked by these meetings was integration with hospitals, and the conditions were ripe: As times and practices were changing for Stern, so were they changing for hospitals: Hospitals were looking to a future defined by ambulatory centers. "Their old way of relying on physicians to bring patients to them was going away," Arie recalls. A realization followed. As Arie puts it, hospitals saw a "need to partner with physicians in a way that guarantees doctors are going to bring their services to them so the hospital can hold onto their ambulatory care." Steven Gubin expands on Arie's observations:

"That's where it was going, for sure. You're measured in so many different ways—length of stay, cost, quality—in order to improve, hospitals and groups have to be on the same page. In the past, everybody worked in silos: Doctors did their thing; hospitals did their thing. The cardiology care has always been superb, but doctors and hospitals didn't understand each other. In order to be a top destination center, however, you have to work together; use the strengths of both."

One of the first initiatives set into motion was a joint venture between Stern and Baptist Memorial Hospital DeSoto. Arie remembers the first meetings, when he told hospital administrators, "We're going to put you guys on the map." Stern moved into the directorship position and Arie's promise was

soon borne out: By 2014, U.S. News & World Report had named Baptist DeSoto the best hospital in the state. "We're the only hospital in Mississippi recognized for cardiology: heart attack outcomes, ICM implementation . . . we turned this place into an entirely different department," Arie says, looking back.

When the partnership was reported publicly in January 2011, Baptist's then-President and CEO, Jim Boswell, was quoted as saying:

"Legally it's an acquisition, but Baptist Memorial Medical Group thinks of it as a partnership. The CEO of Stern (Debbie Eddlestone) is still running the business, but she and I work closely together."

Nearing a decade into the Baptist-Stern collaboration, Steven Gubin continues to share Boswell's view, though he notes that the partnership runs much deeper. "We've been with Baptist the whole time—it's like dating for 90-plus years," Steven likes to joke. In earnest, however, he credits the strength of the relationship to group physicians going back to Neuton Stern, followed by Tom Stern, David Holloway and Jan Turner. "They were always involved, but I think the relationship has gotten even better," Gubin says. Arie agrees, explaining, "We as a group are currently able to provide the level of care that we do because of the relationship we have with the hospital. At the top, our agendas are similar: We are all about delivering great care."

In 2006, Baptist Memorial Health Care Foundation created the Thomas N. Stern, M.D. Award for Excellence in Cardiovascular

Medicine. The award was given at Tom's 80th birthday celebration by Stephen Reynolds.

Debbie Eddlestone thinks it's important to note that Stern's collaboration with Baptist doesn't close the door on patients whose insurance plans are affiliated with other hospitals. "We have always participated in insurance plans despite hospital affiliation," she says, explaining how such a business decision can positively impact patients and enable collaboration with other area hospitals: "Right now, as an example, patients with Cigna health insurance have to go to Methodist. But, Stern can provide services to hospitals in the Methodist Le Bonheur Healthcare system. We provide call coverage and cath coverage; we round there; we do procedures there every day. We still are a fully participating provider."

The collaboration did, however, prompt another name change. The Stern Cardiovascular Center became the Stern Cardiovascular Foundation upon merging with Baptist in 2011.

HEART TRANSPLANTATION

By the time of the merger with Baptist, heart transplantation was nothing new to Stern. The practice pioneered its program in 1985 and in 1993, welcomed Todd Edwards, M.D., as its sole physician focused on transplantation.

Todd came to Stern from the University of Pittsburgh, a major transplant center where he completed residency and a fellowship in cardiology. In retrospect, the prevailing technology of the day was limiting. Consider the left ventricular assist device (LVAD).

Since the first successful implantation of the device in 1966, the LVAD had given life to patients with persistent or severe heart failure symptoms who were awaiting donor hearts, and to those who were not candidates for transplantation. Unlike an artificial heart, the LVAD allows the heart to remain in place; a mechanical pump assists the left ventricle. But even in its second generation, the pump performed the critical function of initiating blood flow. In the new millennium, the technology evolved into its third generation: a dischargeable LVAD in which the pump acts in parallel to the patient's heart.

Todd acknowledges what a game-changer that evolving technology has proven to be—and that technology isn't the only area that's advancing. In 2011, he became Heart Transplantation Program Director for Stern and Medical Director of Heart Transplantation for Baptist. Since that time, Todd and his team have focused on improving the program's structure and capacity to treat patients. The team now numbers 30—a mix of cardiologists, surgeons, a quality manager and physical therapist, among others—with plans to add a fourth cardiologist and a third surgeon. The team is also reporting stronger outcomes than ever.

As Todd acknowledges, the success of Stern's Heart Transplantation Program reflects the practice's age-old goals: to provide unmatched care on a foundation of excellence: "Between St. Louis, Little Rock and Nashville, there's no other place that can do what we can do. We've been doing transplants at Baptist for 34 years, for over 400 patients," he says.

QUALITY AND COMPLIANCE

Colleen LaCroix joined Stern in 2004 as Director of Nursing, but in 2010, she was asked to consider the newly created position of Director of Quality and Compliance. "We knew things were about to start changing," Colleen remembers. Still, she acknowledges, "Our group's initial understanding of how things needed to change occurred when Dr. Stern first pushed for electronic health records—the EHR is the first thing you need to monitor quality."

Exactly what change did Colleen and her colleagues see on the horizon? As she explains it, "Medicare was no longer going to be a passive payer—they were becoming an active purchaser. They wanted to pay for good quality and would incentivize you to do the right things."

In other words, quality would be key. "In this timeframe, we had to look at how we approach care. It couldn't be 20 different doctors approaching the same problem 20 different ways," Arie Szatkowski recalls. In 2011, that led Arie to push for an Institute for Healthcare Improvement (IHI) audit and form an internal Quality Committee.

The first order of business was deciding which metrics to track. As Arie remembers: "We started looking at the patient experience through the journey of coming through the door and leaving," he explains, monitoring how every detail from wait times to the prompt completion of dictations and delivery of test results impacted patient satisfaction. To implement a standard, Stern turned to the tentacle registry that gathers metrics on more than 30 patient contact points.

After defining such baseline metrics, Stern's Quality Committee sparked internal conversations focused on quality. First, it was a conversation among committee members about how to effectively introduce measurement to a group of physicians who were already in the top one percent for productivity and quality in the nation. "We spent a lot of time talking with everyone about what they do, and what they could do, to improve outcomes," Arie remembers. To challenge physicians, the committee created incentives. Pods that showed the highest percentage in reduction of wait times earned a pizza party, for example. "We are constantly challenging our team to do things better," Arie says.

Stern's track record earned Colleen an invitation to speak at the North American College of Cardiology Quality Summit in March 2019. "This was the first year that outpatient data registries were even a part of their national conference," explains Colleen. Today, PINNACLE, the American College of Cardiology's outpatient registry, uses Stern's Quality and Compliance program as its prototype.

Back in the office, Colleen and her team of four work tirelessly with the EHR and Stern physicians to bridge patient care with data reporting. "It's really powerful to see how the data impacts frontline patient care," she notes. But patient registries aren't the only source of data that informs the work of Colleen's team. In 2012, the team implemented a patient satisfaction survey.

The survey asks questions designed to generate feedback around the patient experience in general, and around communication and efficiency, specifically. So far, so good: Stern Cardiovascular Foundation currently scores in the 88th percentile nationally for patient satisfaction. Colleen notes that the survey results are simply a reflection of Stern's corporate culture: "We have the patient at the fore of everything we do," she says. When her team publishes its periodic newsletter for interoffice use, they recognize employees who have been praised in patient surveys, often including the patients' positive words.

While Colleen is quick to note that Stern "has always had quality and compliance at the core," the creation of her team and the joint venture with Baptist amplified the quality of care delivered by both organizations. In one example, Stern shared its experience with outpatient registries to help Baptist improve its performance on inpatient registries.

Currently, Arie leads the Quality Committee for Stern's joint venture with Baptist, which he describes as a "concerted effort by the joint operations, strategic and financial committees, working in tandem with Stern's internal Quality Committee." That committee, in turn, is led by Colleen.

CARDIAC REHABILITATION

Study the history of Stern and Baptist, and you'll discover several successful cases of collaboration. One such case was the launch of Baptist's Cardiac Rehabilitation program out of Stern's main office in Germantown. The program began in 2012. "It was a success-

ful venture," Debbie Eddlestone notes, attributing the success of the program to strong patient and physician engagement. "Our doctors would oversee the program on a daily basis, and be on call for the program," Debbie explains. Patients—in most cases recovering from cardiovascular events or surgery—further benefited from Stern's one-stop shop convenience and simplicity (easy parking!). The physical collaboration ended in 2017 when Baptist made the decision to adopt the standards of the Pritikin Intensive Care Rehabilitation Program. Program standards stipulate that the cardiac rehabilitation program must be housed under the hospital's roof. Today, four Baptist hospitals offer the outpatient program and the collaboration with Stern has evolved in turn: Stern cardiologist Dharmesh Patel, M.D., serves as medical director for the program at Baptist DeSoto.

MERGER WITH MEMPHIS HEART CLINIC

The ripple effect of Stern's collaboration with Baptist touched more than quality and compliance. Engaging on a deeper level with Baptist DeSoto allowed Stern physicians to solidify relationships with Memphis Heart doctors as the groups worked busy, productive days together, foretelling other positive changes to come. In 2012, Stern Cardiovascular Foundation and Memphis Heart Clinic merged.

The merger expanded the practice from 21 to 32 doctors, which helps explain why Stern added another physical location in March 2012 (6027 Wolf River Boulevard in Germantown). "Memphis Heart Clinic was a very successful group.

A lot of the doctors there had at one time been at Stern," Debbie Eddlestone explains, noting that on one level, the merger represented a reunification. But the merger worked on several levels. Objectively, Debbie saw "two great groups," both successful with what they were doing in complementary areas; both practicing in the same hospital system. From that perspective, she saw an opportunity for synergy. "We could make patient care better and cover more," she identified, and so began the process of integrating the two groups.

"Bringing two competing groups together has been a positive for both of us. It made us able to be on the same page; for Baptist, it's a win-win. We saw the big picture and knew we'd be better as one."
—Steven Gubin, M.D.

We would like to recognize the individuals from Memphis Heart Clinic who joined Stern in 2012:

Paul Hess

Steven Himmelstein

David Kraus

Amit Malhotra

Dharmesh Patel

Joseph Samaha

Bashar Shala

Arsalan Shirwany

Jeffrey Kerlan

Stacy Smith

Jiang Cui

Gilbert Zoghbi

Milton B. Addington

David Lan

STRUCTURAL HEART PROGRAM

"Close collaboration is really the best medical care for the patient."
—Basil Paulus, M.D.

With collaboration as the theme of the decade, a new program inside Stern fit right in with the spirit of the era.

Basil Paulus, M.D., joined the group in 2010 as an interventional cardiologist. Around the same time, the advent of structural heart procedures was beginning to transform the cardiovascular world. Stern started its own conversation around building a program in-house, and began looking for the person who would lead it.

Practice leaders approached Basil, who admits, "I was a little scared. I had received little [structural heart] training as a trainee and as a fellow." Yet Basil soon completed specialized training at Columbia University and established Stern's Structural Heart Program in November 2011. The group—the first of its kind in Memphis—performed its first transcatheter aortic valve replacement (TAVR) in February 2012.

Since that time, Basil estimates the group has performed more than 1,000 structural heart procedures, and collaboration is key to each and every one: Procedures truly begin with a weekly conference bringing together Basil's team, interventional cardiologists and cardiovascular surgeons. Each patient's case is considered. Can the patient expect his or her best outcome from drug therapy? An open-heart procedure? A structural heart procedure? The goal of the weekly conference is to explore the best course of treatment for each

patient. "When we leave the conference, we're in 100% agreement. That's why we have the results we have; we do the best thing for the patient," Basil explains.

The collaboration continues as the group heads into the operating room. Depending on the type of structural heart procedure to be performed, personnel will include the surgeon in addition to select members of Stern's Structural Heart team. That might be Dr. Paulus himself or Jay Gardner, M.D.; Joseph Samaha, M.D.; Gilbert J. Zoghbi, M.D., or Paul Hess, M.D., who provides critical invasive imaging during certain procedures. That's what Basil is most proud of. As he shares, "Our program really brings together people from different sub-specialties of cardiology—imaging, intervention, structural heart specialists and also the surgeons—into one group working together to help the patient."

And with more structural heart advances in development, such as protocols for mitral valve replacement and repair, Basil looks forward to evolving Stern's program along with this emerging field of cardiology. "We're doing things now I didn't even dream we'd be doing when we started, helping people we thought were unhelpable," he explains.

WELLNESS AND WEIGHT LOSS CLINIC

If you recall the circumstances surrounding the establishment of Stern's Lipid Clinic, you'll hear echoes in the arc of its Wellness and Weight Loss Clinic. "At Stern, we've been very forthcoming in our preventive medicines," asserts

Debbie Eddlestone, acknowledging the disconnect between prevention and the priorities of our current healthcare system. "It's not an initiative most insurances cover," Debbie acknowledges, despite increasing interest on the part of patients. "We're seeing a lot of patients who want to know, 'How healthy am I?,'" she reports. For some patients, Debbie explains, a professional response to that curiosity can mean catching a problem early to avoid a cardiac event in the future. For others, it can mean delivering critical education about personal cardiac health. For still others, it can be the start of a healthy weight-loss and exercise program.

This desire on the part of patients to take a proactive role in their health grew into Stern Cardiovascular Foundation's Wellness and Weight Loss Clinic in 2014. To participate, a patient must have permission from their established cardiologist. Health coaches staffed by Stern—one full-time and five part-time—counsel patients; Stern cardiologists monitor activity. The ramp-up period requires dedication. "It can be very difficult for patients on multiple medications to feel well enough to start an exercise program," Debbie offers as an example. But the engagement of Stern staff connects patients with tools, starting with a nutrition program. The program is designed to facilitate weight loss, then help patients transition into healthy dietary habits they can sustain for life. "You can have congestive heart failure or diabetes and be on a successful weight-loss plan monitored by your cardiologist. In fact, we've seen patients lose 60 or 70 pounds and come off of their diabetes and cardiology medications," Debbie reports.

Sometimes, she notes, even a small drop in weight is all it takes for a patient to enthusiastically embrace a healthy regime.

Stern has, in fact, begun to stock the pre-packaged, low-carbohydrate snacks that are part of the Wellness and Weight Loss Clinic's nutrition plan. Between the space required for inventory and the fact that new patients are joining every day, Debbie explains, "We hardly market it—we're already outgrowing the space we're in!" With more than 500 participants enrolled since the program's inception, it's no wonder.

A Patient's Perspective: Nell Lingua

Today, if you had the pleasure of meeting Nell Lingua—a crack conversationalist with elegant comportment—you'd never imagine that 10 years ago, she was suffering acutely from an undiagnosed illness. "I was dying," she says matter-of-factly, explaining how her general practitioner referred her to see Steven Gubin. "I had gotten so sick, I was going every place on a cane, then a walker, then in a wheelchair," Nell remembers, though she struggles to recall many other firsthand memories of the time—such was the severity of her illness. A niece who accompanied her to appointments with Steven has since helped Nell fill in some of the details. "Dr. Gubin figured out that I had aortic stenosis. He knows everything," she adds with a wink.

Her niece remembered something else about the diagnosis Steve gave Nell. "You only live two years with that. I was already in my second year," Nell relays.

What Nell does remember clearly is this: A minimally invasive procedure nicknamed TAVI (for transcatheter aortic valve implementation) was a new option. The procedure was, in fact, designed for patients who need valve repair but who are not candidates for open heart surgery due to age or other health problems. The catch? It hadn't caught on—yet—in Memphis. "Steve worked diligently to keep me alive while Basil Paulus and Ed Garrett Jr. learned to do this new surgical procedure," Nell explains. Still, she was cautious. "Dr. Gubin called me after they had successfully completed their first surgery and I asked him to wait a day or two to take me," she smiles. That made Nell patient number 13 to undergo TAVI at Baptist Memorial Hospital Memphis. It was March 2012.

In 2015, a bacterial infection affected Nell's mitral valve, requiring another procedure to attach two mitral valve clips. She likes to joke, "You have four valves in your heart. I have one catheter valve, two clips in my second valve, 60 percent blockage in the third valve and I think the fourth one is okay."

All kidding aside, Nell says she's committed to following her doctors' orders, whether that means switching to decaffeinated coffee or continuing, at least five mornings a week, to perform some of the exercises she's learned in physical therapy through the years. "I am blessed to have such a brilliant team of doctors from Stern. Dr. Gubin calls me a miracle—his 85-year-old poster child," she adds.

If Nell Lingua is Steven Gubin's 85-year-old poster child, consider the story of David Pollow, who

spoke to us through his wife, Pearl. When asked how long David has been a patient of Steven Gubin's, Pearl tweaks her answer just so: "Dr. Gubin has saved my husband's life for at least 10 years," she responds. "Plus, Dr. Gubin made my husband his personal friend," she adds. Pearl likes to tell people that "Dr. Gubin has survived her husband," and even gives Steven credit when it comes to David's longevity. "I'm glad we've had him for a doctor. David is 100 years old and that's part of the help Dr. Gubin has given him," Pearl asserts.

A Portrait of Philanthropy

"To be a great doctor you have to have intellect and humanity. Tom Stern had great humanity. He was devoted to civil rights, human rights and a greater community." —Elissa Fine

On the subject of leading by example, the Stern family's quiet charity set one of the very best.

Early records chronicle the work of Beatrice Stern, wife of Neuton, from serving on the Board of Directors for the Health and Welfare Planning Council of the Memphis Community Fund* (now the United Way) to directing publicity for the American Red Cross during World War II. As Susan Edelman recalls, "My grandmother used to say, 'The order of importance of things is your family, your community and yourself.' That's how you look at the world. That's evidenced in the things my parents and grandparents have done."

For Tom Stern, those deeds ranged from serving on the

board—and for several boards, serving as president or vice president—of the Memphis Arts Council, Opera Memphis, Memphis Orchestral Society, Memphis Brooks Museum of Art and the Community Foundation of Greater Memphis. Together with his wife, Harriet, Tom committed deeply to the local Jewish community and public education: Husband and wife were founding members and presidents of the Jewish Historical Society of Memphis and the Mid-South; Tom also served on the Board of Trustees for Temple Israel and as a member of the National Executive Council of the American Jewish Committee. From 1980 to 1992, Tom sat on the board of Memphis City Schools, serving as president in 1982 and 1986. As his nurse, Randy Meeks remembers those years well: "He decided when he first won that he was going to be very engaged. Every Monday when school was in session, we started rounds later because he would choose a school in town and go to that school early to meet with the principal and teachers and look in on classes. He did it faithfully for all those years."

In its 1993 profile of Tom Stern, The Commercial Appeal quoted Maxine Smith—local education advocate, civil rights leader and Executive Secretary of the NAACP Memphis Branch—as saying, "He is a brilliant person. Whatever he goes about, there is a tenacity. He gives himself completely to the task at hand."

For her part, Harriet Stern chose to seek employment with Memphis City Schools. As Randy recalls, "She was a school teacher and once their kids were grown, she went to the University of

Memphis for her master's degree and taught at one of the poorest schools in town, LaRose Elementary." Before retiring in 1989, Harriet would teach at White Station Elementary School as well. Elissa Fine, Stern's Lipid Clinic Coordinator and a personal friend of Harriet, shared this remembrance:

"Harriet was all over this town helping kids to read. A woman once told me she came to an appointment with a friend because her friend said she was going to the Stern office. The woman had said to herself, 'I wonder if that's Mrs. Stern who taught me in high school?' She wanted to tell me how Mrs. Stern was always encouraging her. She told me, 'I am where I am today because of her.'"

While it's easy to imagine that Harriet would have warmed hearing this personal testimony, those who observed her knew one thing unequivocally: "She wanted no public recognition. She did it because it was what you do," Randy asserts. Steven Gubin notes the same of Tom Stern: "He did so much for the city. You wouldn't know a lot of it, probably, because he didn't care about [the recognition]." As Elissa Fine puts it, "They didn't live on the golf course. They lived for the people."

When Harriet Stern passed away in 2012, her eulogy referenced tikkun olam, a Jewish concept of repairing the world through acts of kindness. For Harriet and Tom, the concept infused their personal and professional lives. "The Sterns were helpful and community-driven. A part of that got woven into the clinic silently," explains Jennifer Morrow. James Klemis agrees: "There's a genuine love for

the community inside Stern—it's always been a service-oriented group."

Frank McGrew remembers an early example: "Tom was very interested in getting care for minorities. He went out of his way to help them any way he could. He looked after some prominent African American patients and was friends with African American doctors who referred their patients to him."

In the aftermath of September 11, 2001, the practice reached out to local police and fire personnel. "We were open on a Saturday; we didn't charge anything. We did stress testing and checkups on anyone who was a first responder," remembers Sharon Goldstein.

Years later, Stern employees learned that Memphis' sanitation workers—whose safe and equitable working conditions brought the Rev. Dr. Martin Luther King Jr. to the city, and to his assassination, in 1968—remained underserved. "It started conversations when we found out that the sanitation workers had never gotten what Martin Luther King wanted them to get, which was a pension. So they work until they just can't work anymore. We got together with then-Mayor A C Wharton and reached out. Dr. Gubin and I went; one time, Dr. Szatkowski and I went—to tell them who we were and how we wanted to help them. We went to their job sites where they report every morning and we would give free cardiac screenings. It was very rewarding," Debbie says—proof that the memories and lessons of the Sterns' leadership-by-example continue to inspire acts of community healing from within the practice.

Pam Glover remembers Stern engaging in other community initiatives, from feeding the homeless at Memphis Union Mission to coordinating health fairs in the name of prevention. But the spirit of generosity directed inward toward the practice resonates greatly with her, and with several others interviewed for this book. "No matter how big we've gotten, Stern has always had the community of family," Pam says, recalling times when Stern employees quietly took up money for co-workers in need. Other times, she remembers Tom Stern giving a ride to an employee between the office and the bus stop. Other employees recounted stories of the practice's generosity through periods of personal hardship. "That's what we do," Pam offers in explanation.

The practice has also long been involved in philanthropy specific to the specialty of cardiology—dating to 1948 when Neuton Stern himself established the Memphis Heart Association. In 1993, Jan Turner served as President of the West Tennessee Chapter of the American Heart Association. "We had a wonderful group of volunteers and other dedicated individuals. As far as medical charities are concerned, I think the American Heart Association is absolutely tops. Their administrative costs are low and funds are directed toward the appropriate areas," Jan says. Indeed: At the time of this book's publication, the American Heart Association ranked as one of Charity Navigator's 4-Star Charities with a Platinum Seal of Transparency from GuideStar.

Sharon Goldstein echoes Jan Turner when considering Stern's history with the charitable organization. "The AHA has long been a favorite charity of Stern and many of us have been active on all of their fundraisers, educational committees and more. I believe they would call us one of their strongest partners," she says. Undoubtedly: Following in the tradition of Neuton and Tom Stern and Jan Turner, Stern's current leadership remains highly engaged in local AHA initiatives. Steven Gubin, who serves on the Board of Directors for the AHA's Mid-South Chapter, will serve as honorary chairman of the organization's Memphis Heart Ball in 2020; Debbie Eddlestone chaired the organization's 2019 Heart Walk. More than 100 employees of Stern Cardiovascular Foundation participated in and/or contributed to the 2019 Heart Walk, raising $100,000, the practice's highest total to date.

*Another pillar of the Memphis community served on this board with Beatrice Stern: Jack Belz. Jack later became a patient of Tom, and then of Steve Gubin.

A Special Chapter in Philanthropy: The University of Tennessee Health Science Center

In the oral history Neuton and Beatrice Stern gave to the University of Memphis in 1968, Neuton shared a glimpse into the formative years of the institution we know today as the University of Tennessee Health Science Center College of Medicine. In summary:

In the first decade of the 20th century, there were, at most, three private medical schools in our region. These were, in Neuton's words, "combined with the-then University of Tennessee Medical School, a small school in Nashville which was moved to Memphis."

By the early 1920s, Neuton explains:

"There was a proposal because things had gone bad, evidently, during the war. The school had deteriorated and gotten smaller. When there was very considerable discussion as to whether the school should be let go and dissolved I was present at one of the faculty meetings when this problem was discussed. The Medical faculty decided not to be in favor of the dissolution [ensuring that] Memphis doctors would cooperate if the school went on—which it did."

In this way, clinical professor of medicine Neuton Stern helped to secure the future of the fledgling University of Tennessee Medical School.

Later in the same oral history, Beatrice Stern adds:

"The Heart Association and the University of Tennessee together set up a visiting lectureship—professorship—in [Neuton's] name to which any friends or former pupils made donations. This money is used to bring an outstanding man in the field of internal medicine, usually in cardiology, to Memphis. This man may not only give a public lecture, but he is also used during the entire day to work with residents, interns, students and professors from early in the morning until late at night, and Dr. Stern founded it. It is a very nice thing, because it's this sort of thing that's done and then remembered, and Neuton has been able to enjoy three of the Neuton Stern visiting professors, and we hope that we'll enjoy many more."

The endowment Beatrice spoke of was established on the occasion of Neuton's 75th birthday in 1965.

You may recall from Chapter 3 of this book that Tom Stern felt his original calling from the world of academia. We know where his professional path ultimately led, though, like his father before him, Tom made time for teaching—at his alma mater, the school his father had helped to save. Tom even earned a plaque for distinguished teaching as a clinical Professor of medicine (also like his father) at the UTHSC College of Medicine.

The family's deep commitment to the institution inspired a generous gift in 1992, when Tom and Harriet Stern endowed the Neuton S. Stern Professorship in Cardiovascular Diseases. Like its namesake, any candidate for the position must be a "teacher, researcher and clinician."

The Sterns' gift continues giving, perhaps in some unexpected ways. James Klemis remembers how learning of the professorship influenced his decision to join the practice. "The head of Cardiology at the University of Tennessee Medical School was named for Neuton Stern even though this wasn't a private practice," he marvels. To James, this signaled that the practice he was being recruited by presented an opportunity to work within a unique hybrid model.

Today, the work of developing a job description and qualifications for the professorship, along with selecting the appointee, is divided among the Dean and Chancellor of the UTHSC College of Medicine and an advisory committee. Appointments are made for an unspecified period of time, but are not considered lifetime appointments. The current appointee, Karl T. Weber, M.D., was recruited in 1999 from the University of Missouri-Columbia, where he served as Director of the Division of Cardiology. His curriculum vitae cites his clinical and research interest in congestive heart failure and prolific authorship, with more than 550 publications.

Tom and Harriet's tradition of giving to the UTHSC College of Medicine would not end with the professorship. The Stern Merit Endowment is offered to incoming medical students. Jada Williams, Assistant Vice Chancellor for Development Services at UTHSC, notes that recipients must demonstrate "scholastic ability and dedication to medicine as a career," and that the scholarship was "written specifically for African American first-year students." If no applicants fit these criteria, applicants of other ethnicities are eligible. In recent years, Jada reports, two to three recipients annually have benefited from the endowment.

While the Sterns were major boosters of the University of Tennessee, they didn't overlook the University of Memphis, proving their devotion to citywide progress and scholarship. When Tom celebrated his 80th birthday in 2006, the couple established the Thomas N. Stern, M.D., Fund for Excellence in Cardiovascular Medicine, a scholarship benefiting pre-med "Tigers."

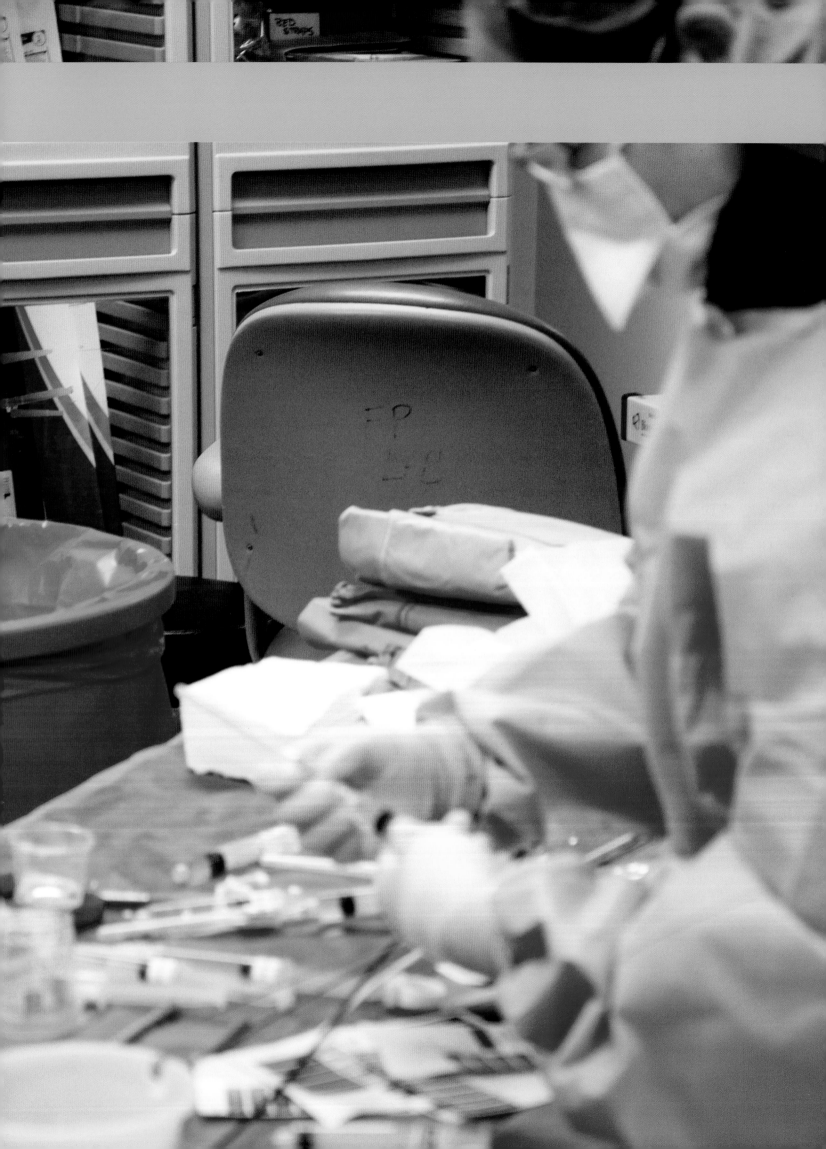

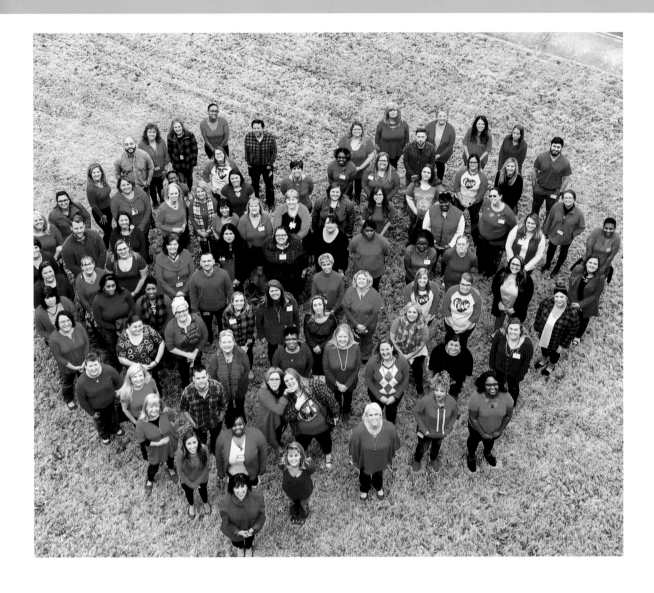

I KNOW THAT ALL OF US CANNOT WORK TOGETHER FOREVER, BUT I KNOW THAT EVERY-
ONE CAN COME TO WORK HERE APPRECIATING THE OPPORTUNITIES THE GROUP'S FOUND-
ERS HAVE GIVEN US." —DAVID HOLLOWAY, M.D., STERN CARDIOVASCULAR FOUNDATION

Ask any employee of Stern Cardiovascular Foundation what the group's second century holds and you'll hear a variety of smart, ambitious answers. Yet behind every response, a common chord resonates: honoring the legacy built by Drs. Neuton and Thomas Stern. (Ask Steven Gubin what the future holds, and you can almost hear Tom's voice in his answer: "I'm proud of what we've accomplished, but we can always continue to improve.")

Employees like Randy Meeks who had the opportunity to work alongside Tom Stern note that his legacy continues to guide the group's journey. "Even though he's been gone since 2006, everything goes back to him," Randy explains, adding, "He had a lot of foresight as to what was coming."

If Tom Stern were alive today, he might see what Arie Szatkowski sees: a healthcare system charac-terized by spiraling costs, inconsis-tent patient outcomes and a trend toward insurance companies and employers—not patients—decid-ing where patients will be seen. On the flipside, he might see the opportunity Arie sees: to set inter-nal targets as a means to achieve national recognition for outstand-ing metrics on outcomes, quality

◀◀ Operations at Baptist
Photo by Stephanie Norwood

◀ Stern staff
Photo courtesy of Stern Cardiovascular Organization

and cost of care delivered—restoring influence over choice and care to Stern patients and physicians, respectively.

Amit Malhotra sees the group's outreach efforts as critical practice for navigating the future. Where cancer care has already gone, cardiac care is headed: discharging hospital patients the same or next day to be managed by home-based care. The paradigm lessens expenses, of course, but also complications, as patients have demonstrated better outcomes recovering in their home environment. "The more outreach we have, the more available we will be to partner with home healthcare agencies [to this end]," Amit explains.

While Stern physicians have always kept a hand in academia—from hosting residents to filling professorial posts—Debbie Eddlestone sees an academic component crystalizing. Specifically, obtaining credentials for the practice as a teaching facility. Amit Malhotra explains that the group is further poised to launch such an initiative through its participation in conferences and lectures at local, national and international levels. As for what the teaching itself might look like? Amit imagines rotating fellowships that would offer specialized training to state-side recruits or international candidates who could take knowledge gained at Stern back to a developing country. Perhaps a training module could be developed to expose local primary care physicians and nurse practitioners to aspects of cardiology currently overlooked by traditional training programs.

"We want to be a center of excellence. It's the idea of leaving something behind—to be stronger than when we first came in, so the practice is strong for another 100 years." —Steven Gubin, M.D.

While Stern team members like Amit outline individual initiatives, Debbie stays focused on the executive dashboard. "We're creating a well-rounded picture. We have the research. Dr. Malhotra has the vision for the academic piece. We've set ourselves in the communities in the tri-state area. At the end of the day, that's something we're really proud of," she says, reviewing the fundamentals Stern will continue to grow on. Steven Gubin acknowledges that Stern's foundation is unique—and full of opportunity. "We have the benefits of a private practice where Debbie can run the day-to-day, with the nature of an academic center where everybody sub-specializes. And we have a good partner in Baptist. Over the last couple of years, there's been movement toward a much more collegial relationship between physicians and hospitals. Continuing to demonstrate that doctors work well with hospital administrators would be a good legacy," he says.

Bringing Stern into its second century will undoubtedly require a balance of staying nimble and staying true to the practice's core values. It will require continual monitoring of the changing healthcare ecosystem and Stern's place within it. Arie's outlook is confident: "Healthcare continues to evolve. We are always thinking about how we navigate the changes going on around us. But the reason we've survived so long is because we've stayed together, like a family that has disputes. We've always managed to work them out

and come out on top. We're at our best when we're together."

To that point, Stern will keep one thing constant as it moves into its second century: valuing the unique contributions of doctors across the spectrum.

As Jennifer Morrow explains, "Cardiology is a field that moves fast. At the same time, there is a large part of cardiology that depends on a lifetime of experience; there are some diseases you may see once in a career. We get the benefit of being fluent in new technology from our young guys while having this encyclopedic knowledge of the careers of our older guys. Not all groups have that and it's like the loss of a culture without it—no more of that oral or written tradition."

That tradition is honored at Stern. As this book was in its final stages of development, the group celebrated David Holloway's 50th year of practice while welcoming three new doctors, creating a total of 350 employees across 17 locations in three states—a legacy, indeed.

In addition to nine outreach locations in Arkansas, Mississippi and Tennessee, Stern Cardiovascular Foundation operates eight physical locations. Beyond the main facility in Germantown, these locations include Collierville, East Memphis, Munford and Union City in the state of Tennessee. Mississippi operations include Oxford and two locations in Southaven.

LOOKING BACK ON LEADERSHIP

In 1991, the Tennessee Medical Association Board of Trustees presented its Distinguished

Service Award to Tom Stern. The award recognizes contributions or achievements made during the award year; in Tom's case, inspiring public service.

While strong leadership has been a cornerstone of Stern Cardiovascular Foundation since its inception, there's a reason to consider it near the conclusion of this book.

There are infinite permutations of leadership styles, some with their own mottos and posters. And then there are quiet leaders. Those who lead by doing, setting an example, building consensus—and inspiring others in the process. These leaders don't telegraph their work via mottos or posters; the stories of their lives serve as the reflection.

Taken together, the stories held within this book reflect just that: a line of leaders, dating back to Neuton Stern, who have quietly and humbly provided both model and inspiration. You can see it reflected in Tom Stern's decision to pursue medicine professionally. "His parents never pushed him into medicine," Randy Meeks says. Rather, she learned through the years, Tom Stern made his career decision "because of the way he felt about his father. He had great respect for him. The thing he admired most about Neuton Stern was his equanimity. That was something he inherited from his father and he practiced it," Randy explains.

Similarly, Steven Gubin continues to draw inspiration from Tom Stern. "He didn't talk a lot," Steven remembers of working alongside Tom. Yet, he adds, "If you just watched him, you learned a lot. What I do today is a reflection on him and his father. I often

ask myself, 'What would Dr. Stern do?'"

That mantra has influenced Steven's tenure as President of Stern Cardiovascular Foundation since 2008. "I'm the fourth President, and two were Sterns," he says with a smile, giving a glimpse into the upbeat, easygoing nature that colors his personal leadership style. "I call him the glue that holds this whole group together," Debbie Eddlestone shares, adding, "He is well-loved." Others hold similar views of Debbie herself, whose CEO of the Year distinction from Inside Memphis Business bolsters Stern's tradition of strong leadership. "She's like our mother," Arie Szatkowski says, explaining, "I don't think there's anybody that has the skill—the tenacity—to manage and keep in line a group of complex, highly functioning personalities like she does." Colleen LaCroix sees a continuity in Stern's line of leadership: "Debbie, Dr. Gubin and Dr. Holloway seem to keep Tom Stern at the front of their minds," she observes.

Perhaps there's no better qualified voice on leadership in the Memphis area than Arnold E. Perl: past Chairman of the Memphis-Shelby County Airport Authority, founding Chairman of the Japan-America Society of Tennessee, Chairman Emeritus (Co-Chair) of the Southeast US/Japan Association and co-author of Simple Solutions: Harness the Power of Passion and Simplicity to Get Results, a leadership tome written with Tom Schmitt of FedEx, published in 2006 by John Wiley & Sons, Inc. As established previously in this book, Mr. Perl is also a Stern Cardiovascular Foundation patient. Upon learn-

ing of this publication, he shared the following reflection:

"Stern Cardiovascular Foundation is highly acclaimed not only in the Mid-South, but nationally. It is continuing the strong culture created by the late Neuton Stern and his son Tom Stern, and carried on by the current group of leading physicians and staff. The leadership of Stern today is outstanding in its own right, starting with the strong management style of Dr. Steven Gubin, himself a world-class cardiologist. Memphis is so fortunate that the Stern Cardiovascular Foundation has been a hallmark of preferred cardiology care in the greater Memphis community and surrounding areas in the Mid-South. I expect because of the strong culture, future generations of physicians who come to practice at Stern can continue to be influenced by what the patient community has come to expect: superb care, committed physicians and caring about their fellow man."

Arnold Perl's words seem as fitting a segue as any to these final words from Tom Stern:

"In retrospect, the changes in medicine and the change in practice has been hard to believe. We started from a small office on the second floor of the physicians and surgeons building of the hospital, including two consultation rooms and two examining rooms, and grew up to the current, well-equipped building. I will always be thankful for the privilege of working in such a wonderful environment and to help so many patients. Few people are fortunate enough to enjoy their work as much as I have. Even more wonderful has been the opportunity to be surrounded by a wonderful group of workers and physicians. Few are so privileged."

And yet, the "few" Tom spoke of has grown from one man to 430 employees, from one century to the next, by adapting to change while remaining unchanged in the pursuit of quality and excellence. Time-proven and forward-looking: It's the Stern way.

Outtakes

Over the course of 21 months and interviews with more than 45 individuals, a great volume of oral histories were gathered for this book project. Not all of the quotes were woven into the narrative, though several are comedic, poignant or telling enough to stand on their own. We hope you enjoy them.

On each other, and patients

"There is a camaraderie of sharing the burden of care within our group." —Amit Malhotra

"At Stern, the doctors are teaching everyone constantly, so everyone is as capable as they can possibly be." —Elissa Fine

"Our doctors blow me away with how intelligent they are and how they've dedicated their lives to their jobs. It makes it easier for me. I've sacrificed a lot for the job, but it's a decision I made. I wouldn't have made it if I didn't believe in these doctors." —Debbie Eddlestone

"He always loved his patients and his patients loved him." —Nancy Cummings on Jan Turner

"He has a huge heart and incredible intellect. He never stands in one place at all. If you ask him a question, you're going to go walking around with him." —Elissa Fine on Frank McGrew

"No matter how busy Dr. Russo was, he would sit down with patients, talk and have them laughing. Dr. Holloway would always keep his smile. I was young when I started [at Stern]. Seeing the doctors' kindness bled into how I wanted to be as a person. They taught me to be kind." —Pamela Burks

"You hear patients talk about David Holloway like they would a father." —James Klemis

"When I got married, 65 people from the office came to our wedding. We weren't just employees of an office, we were family. Dr. Holloway gave me away." —Kathy Gwinn

"This man was the same yesterday, today and tomorrow: a good, kind, compassionate person." —Nancy Hardin on Neuton Stern

"I don't care what you call your 'good book' but if you get all the good word out of it, that was Dr. Neuton and Dr. Tom." —Nancy Hardin on Neuton and Tom Stern

"He was quite the character: a man of few words, but whatever words he spoke, you listened very closely." —Scot Feury on Tom Stern

"You stood taller and walked straighter in his presence. He was so soft-spoken but so strong, and yet so kind." —Colleen LaCroix on Tom Stern

"Some people said Dr. Stern was like his name [but] he was soft-spoken; he never raised his voice." —Randy Meeks on Tom Stern

"Although some people saw my father as a very serious kind of guy, there were a few people who saw him as a total softie. Like Garfield's teddy bear, some people called him 'Pookie' behind his back." —David Stern on Tom Stern

"I had the pleasure of working with Dr. Stern. I didn't have to work closely with him, but he was a super-sweet man. He did not give hugs out too terribly often, so when he hugged somebody, everybody took notice." —Melissa Reaves

"He was the epitome of what you wanted a physician to be. It was a luxury and a privilege to work for him." —Judy Jackson on Tom Stern

"He read all the time and kept up with things. One day this drug rep came up and asked to see Dr. Stern. He said okay. She came in and said, 'Thank you for seeing me. I want to talk to you about my drug.' And he said, with a smile, 'You have three minutes to tell me something about your drug that I don't already know.'" —Randy Meeks on Tom Stern

"I like to be busy so I cleaned an exam room one day and felt that someone was watching me. It was Dr. Stern, who said, 'This pleases me so much . . . my mother was the ultimate cleaner!'" —Randy Meeks on Tom Stern

"One of my favorite articles hung on the wall in his office: an article about his father being one of the first people to adopt the ECG. There was another local figure in healthcare quoted as saying, 'We're never going to learn anything from the ECG . . .' Sometimes when I would come into meet with Dr. Stern, I'd go over the article. He would come in and give me his little smile, as though that article was one of his favorite things, too." —Dan Caldwell on Tom Stern

"I have said many times: Dr. Stern was the best boss I ever had, and it still holds true. I became deeply fond and respectful of him . . . he was one in a million." —Dan Caldwell on Tom Stern

"Everything he did, he did very well. He was a regular man who happened to be a doctor. Because of his leadership and the foundation he set for Stern, he made it one of the top-notch places. But the way he felt about people . . . he took the time to learn everyone's name, so when you passed down the hall he knew who you were." —Pam Glover on Tom Stern

On getting to, and staying at, Stern

"We didn't even have a maternity policy when I was pregnant with my first child, but my children have grown up at Stern. I have patients who say, 'I feel like your kids are my grandkids!' You really get to know your patients here." — Jennifer Morrow

"The reason I'm here is that one of my professors told me when I left that I should talk to Dr. Holloway. I bet Holloway is ready for a new partner about now." —Frank McGrew

"I grew up here." —Sharon Goldstein

"Do you remember the karaoke Christmas party? All of us remember how much we loved Dr. Turner's impersonation of Robert Palmer's 'Addicted to Love.' How I love this place. That's why I haven't retired—it's my family." —Nancy Cummings

"We are here to serve—that's the passion of it. I think that's why I've stayed here so long." —Colleen LaCroix

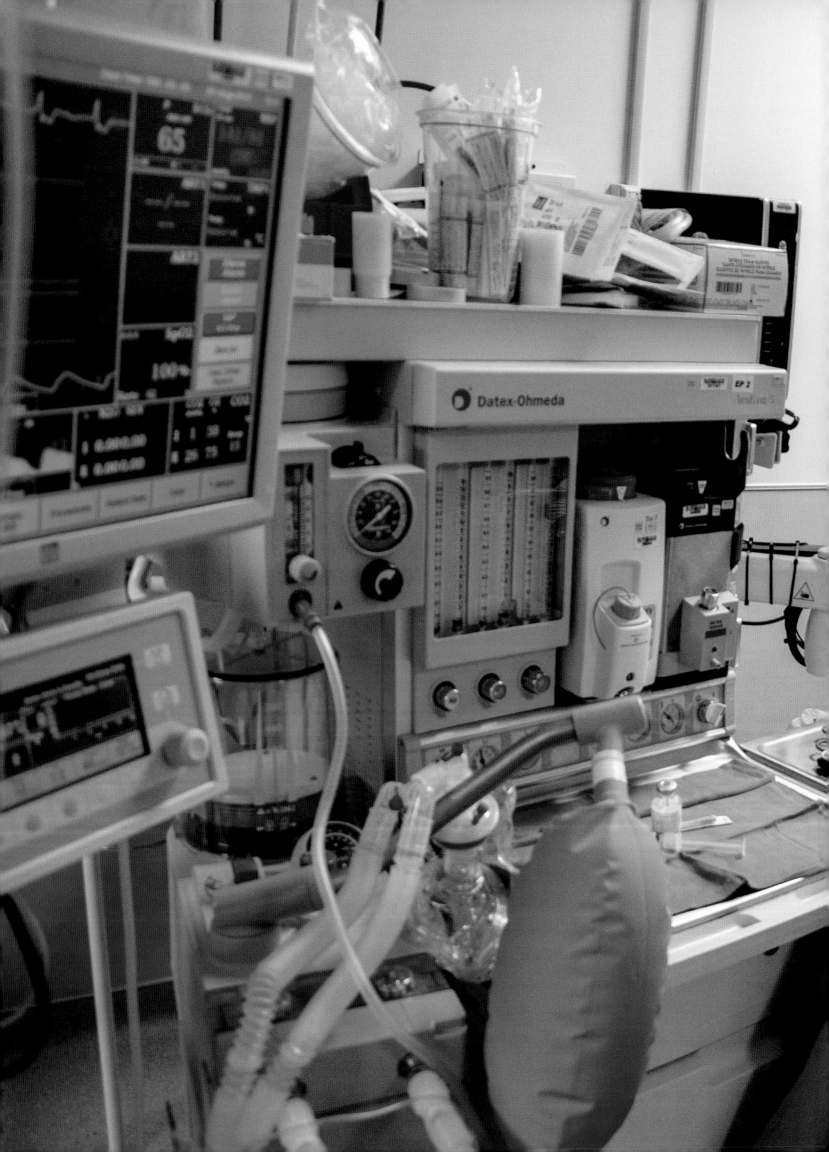

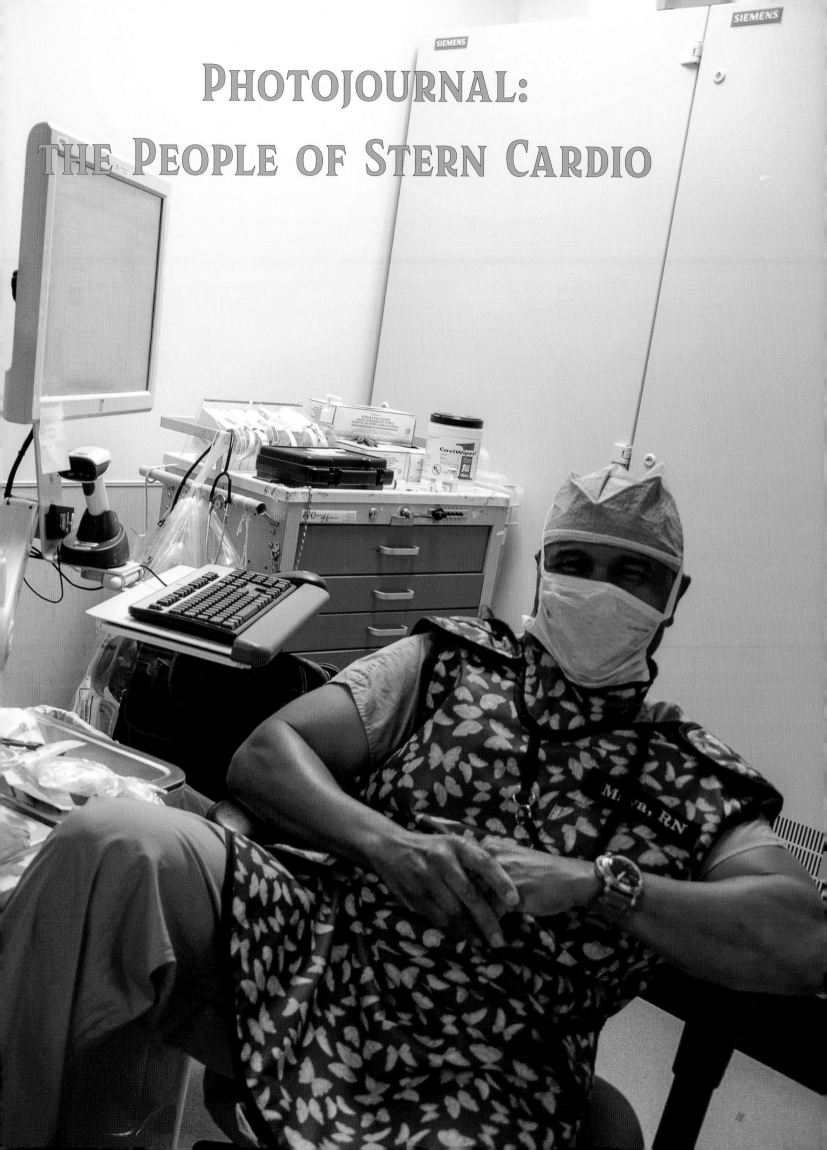

Photojournal:
The People of Stern Cardio

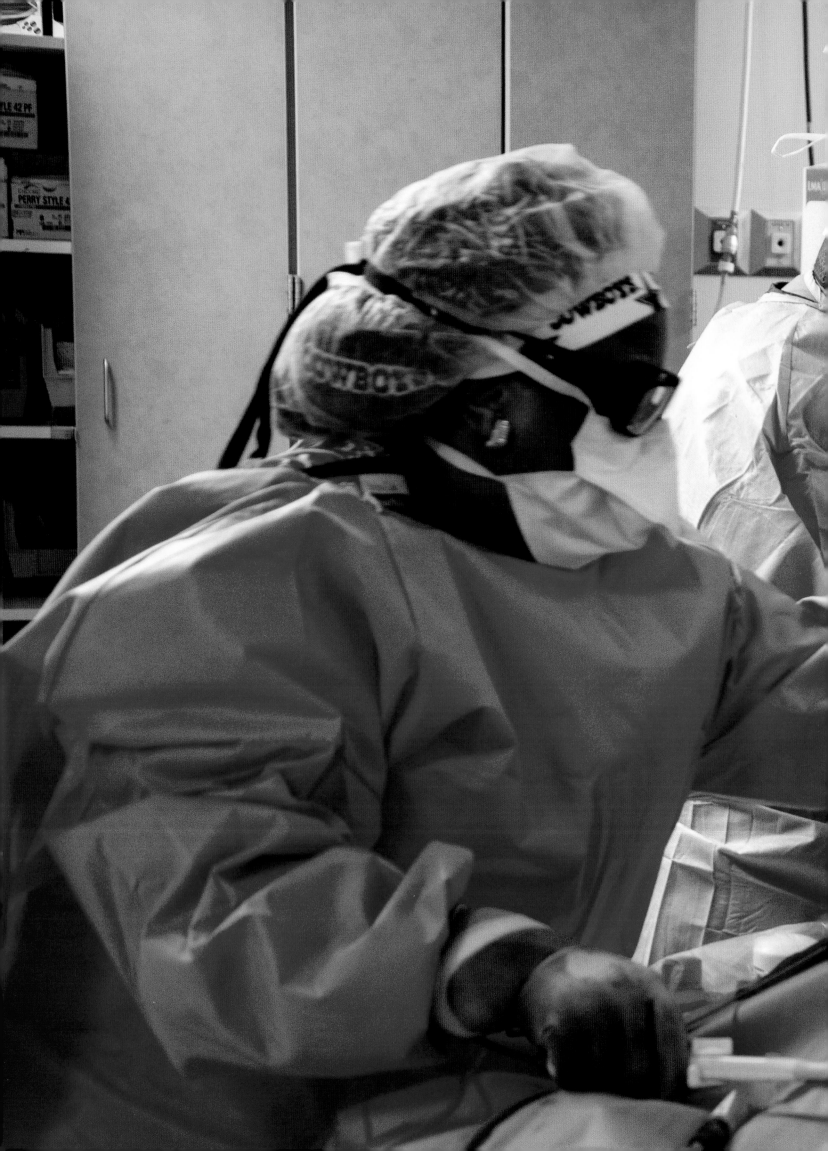

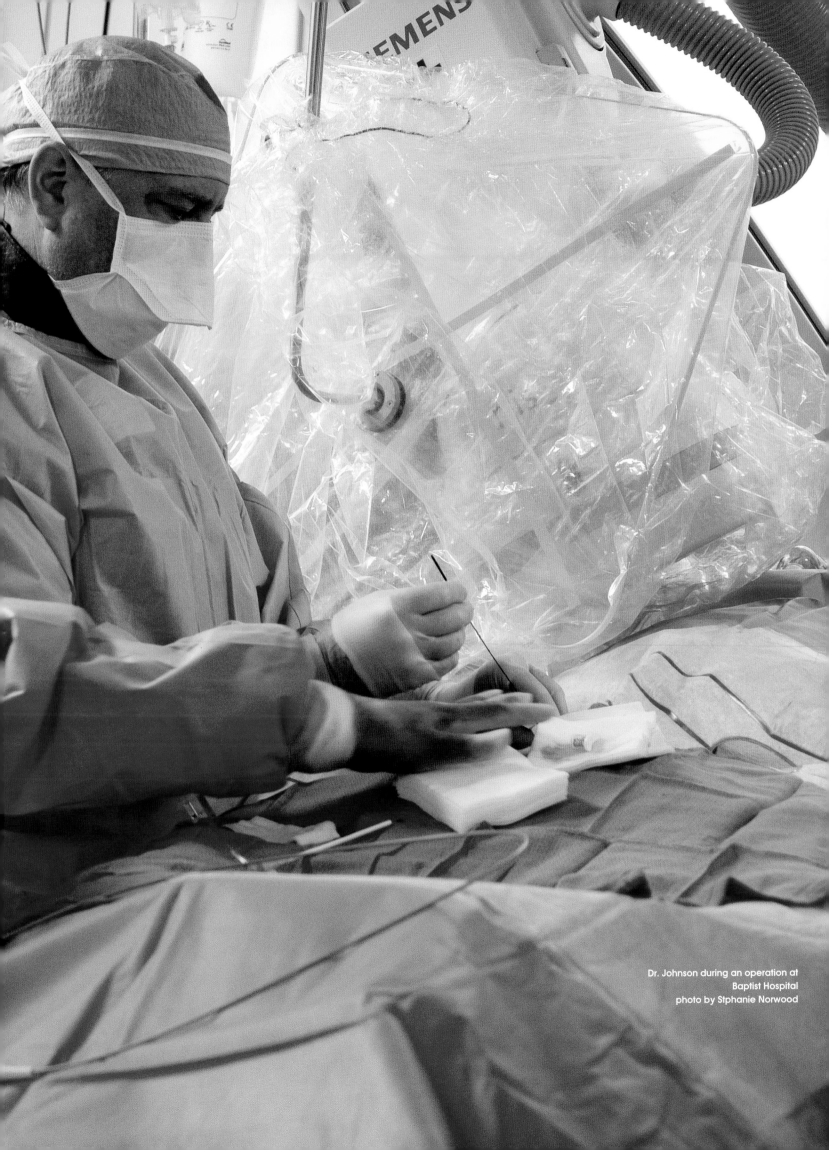

Dr. Johnson during an operation at
Baptist Hospital
photo by Stphanie Norwood

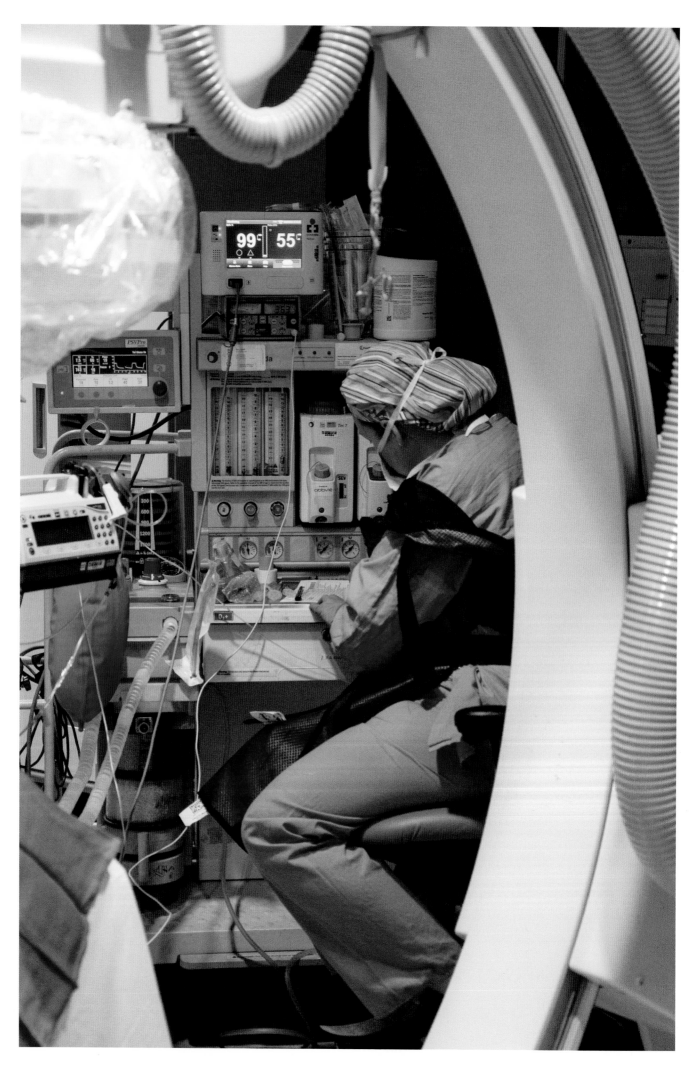

STERN CARDIOVASCULAR FOUNDATION

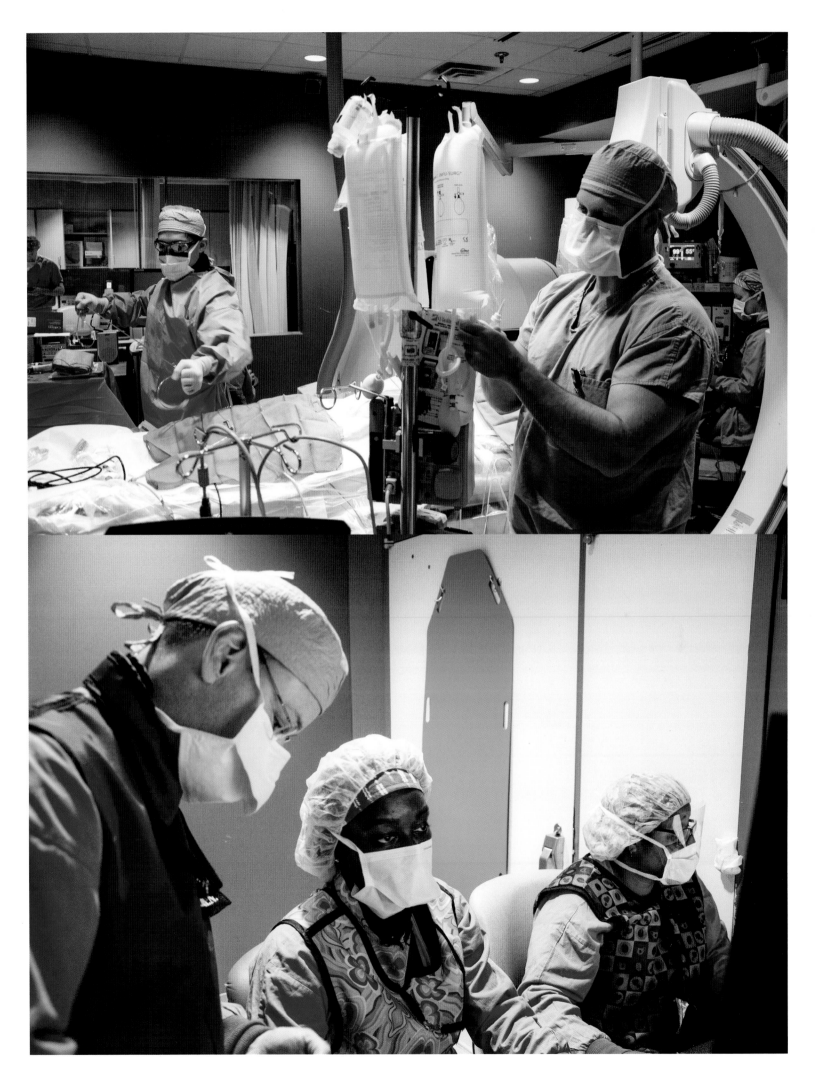

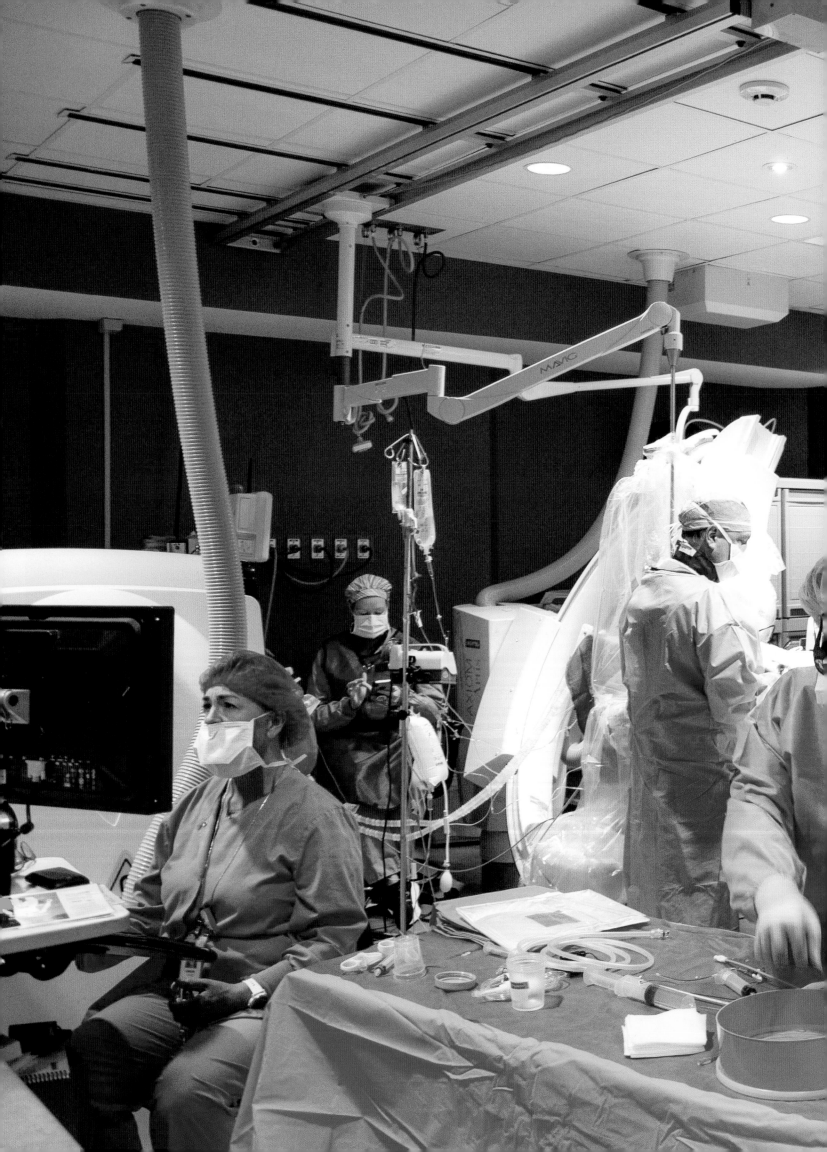

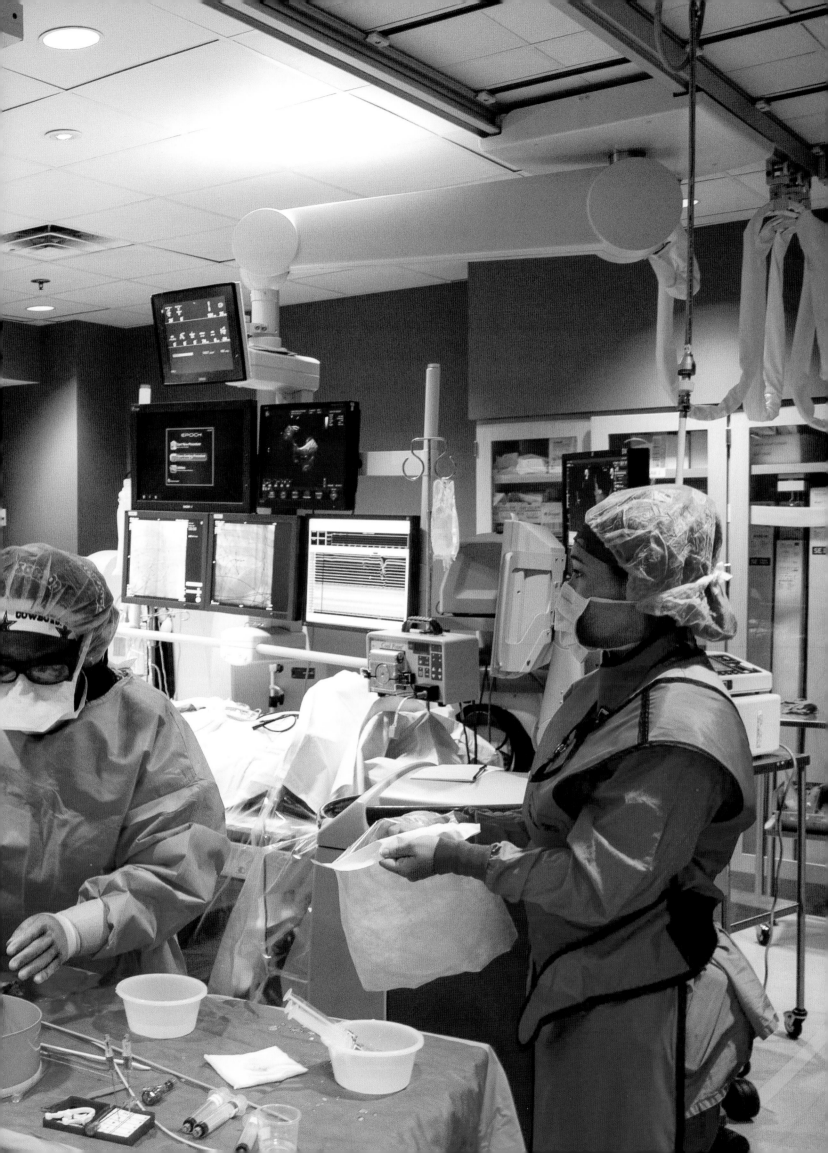

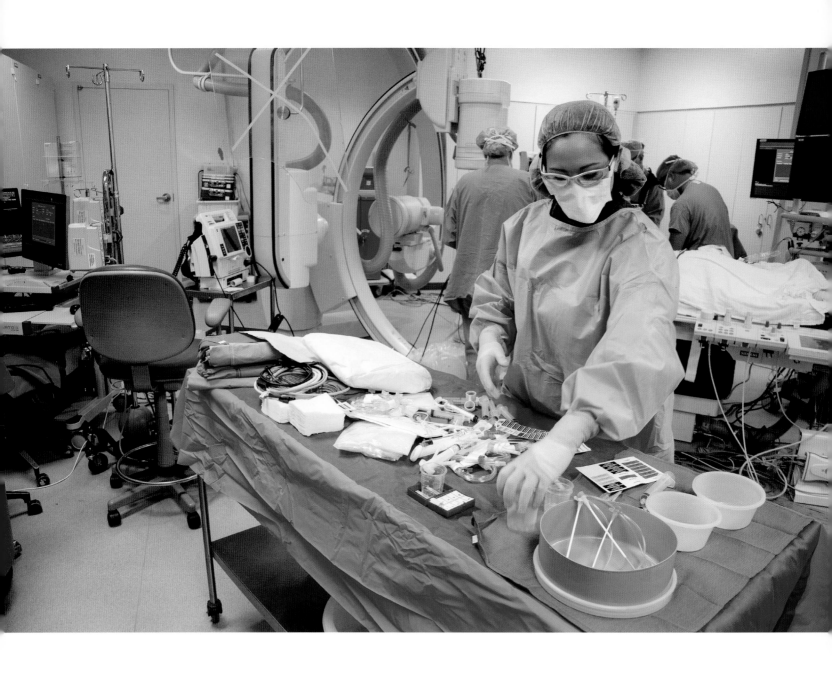

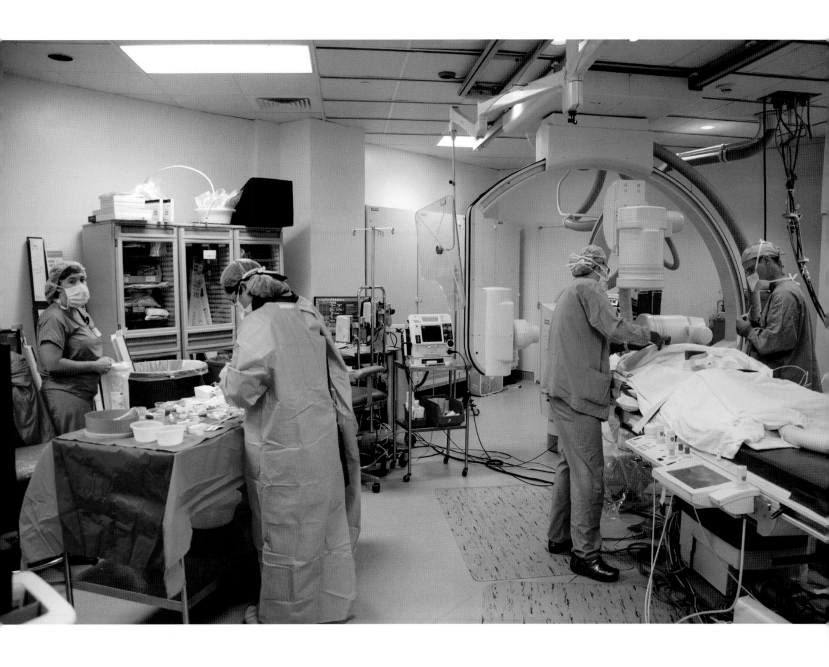

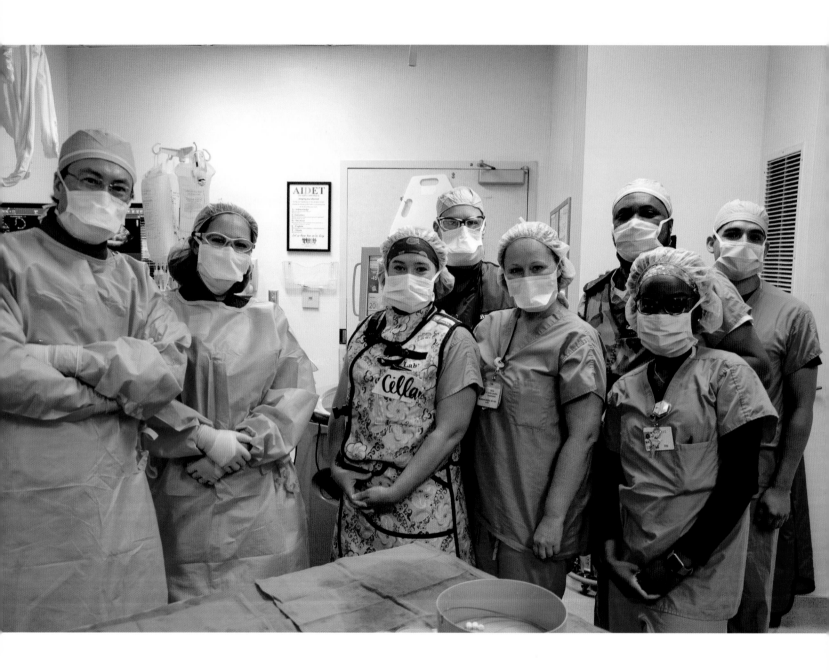

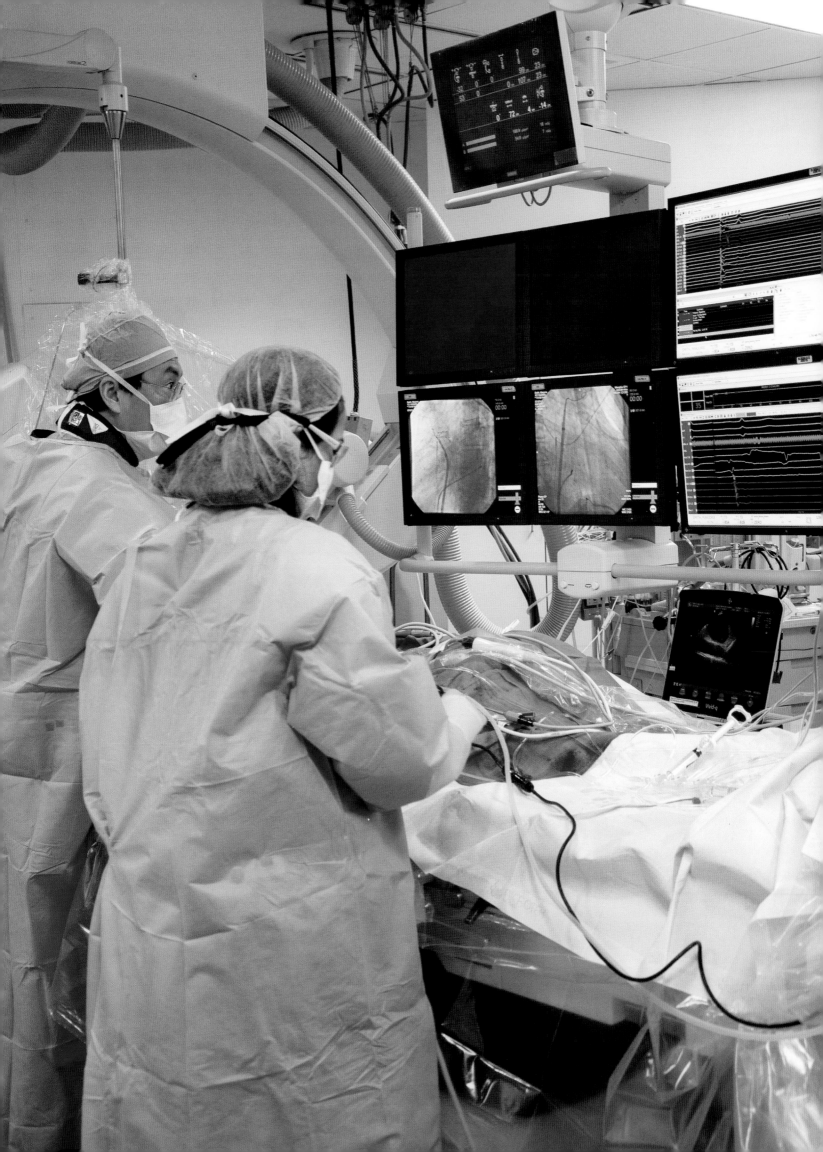

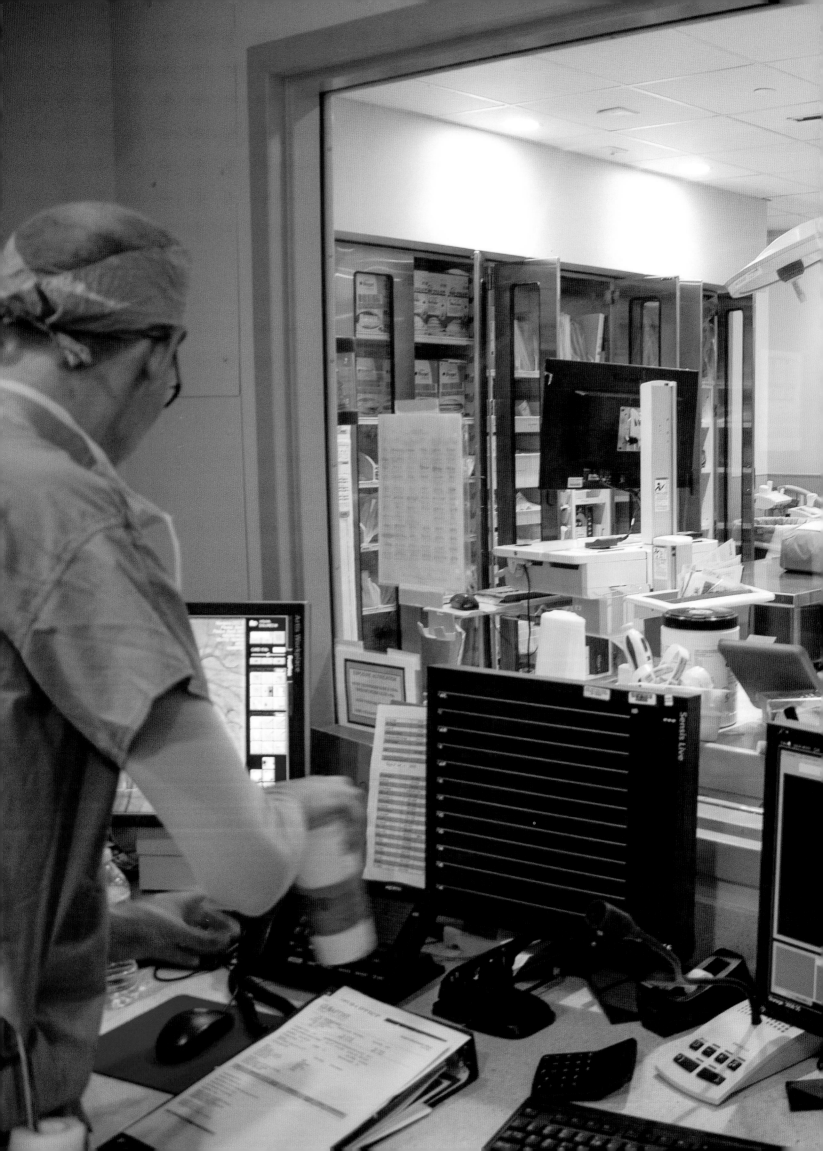

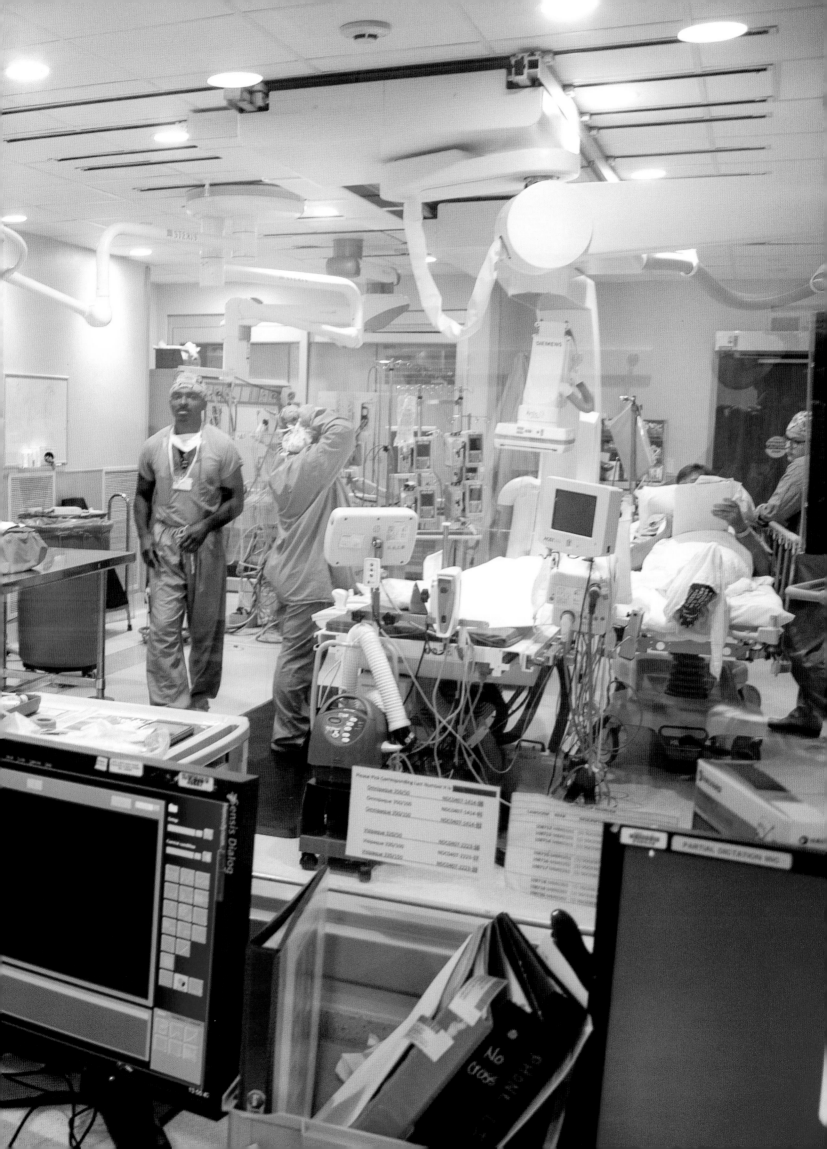

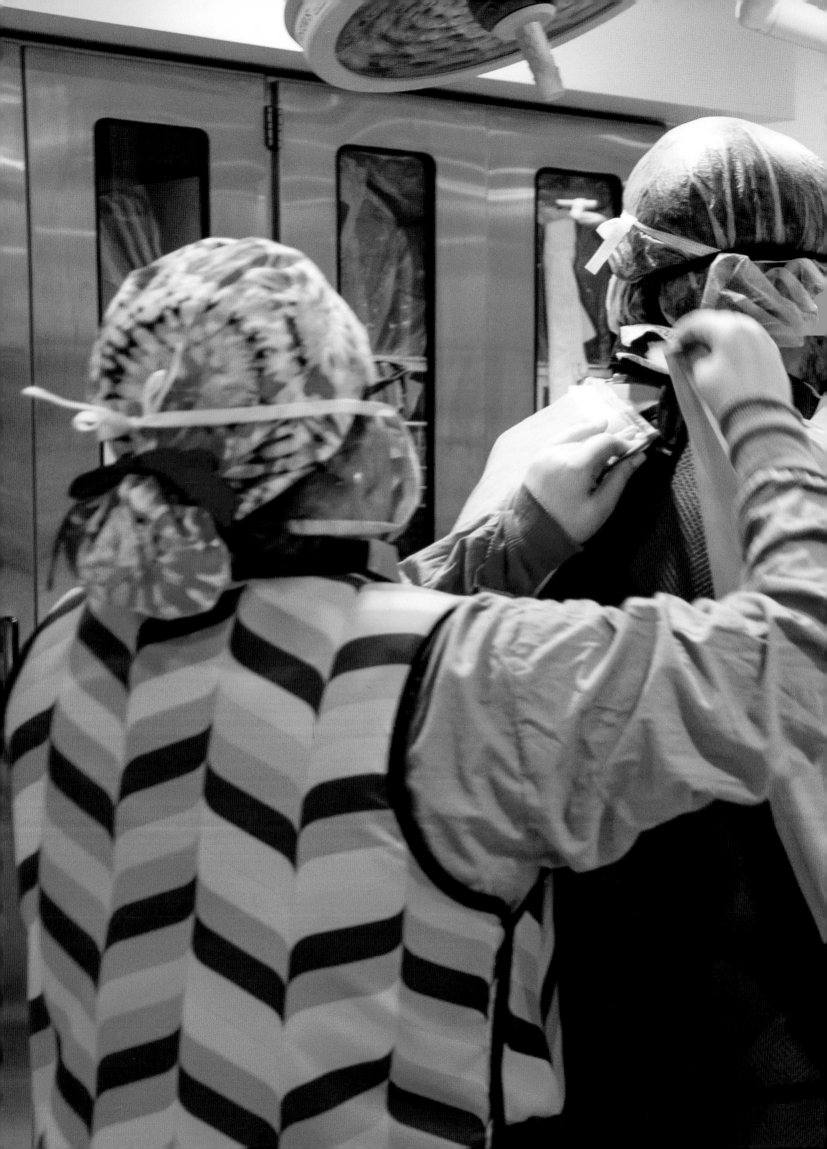

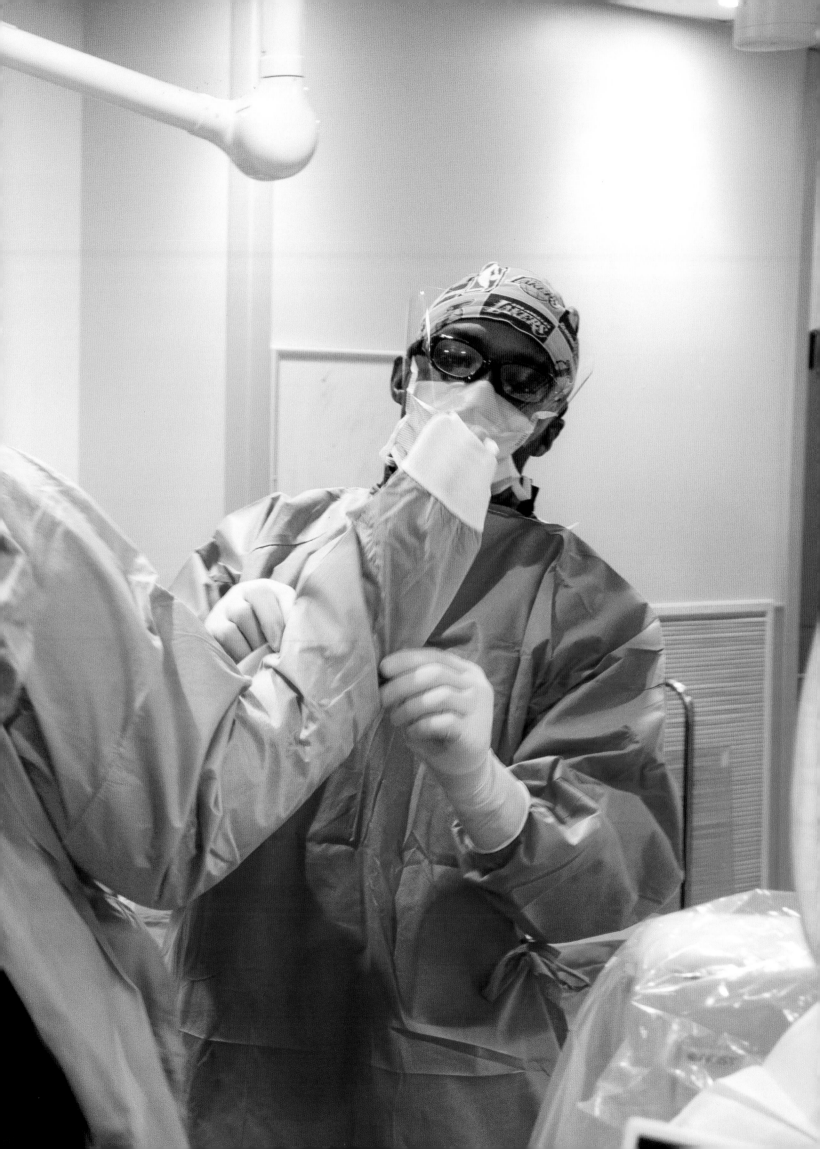

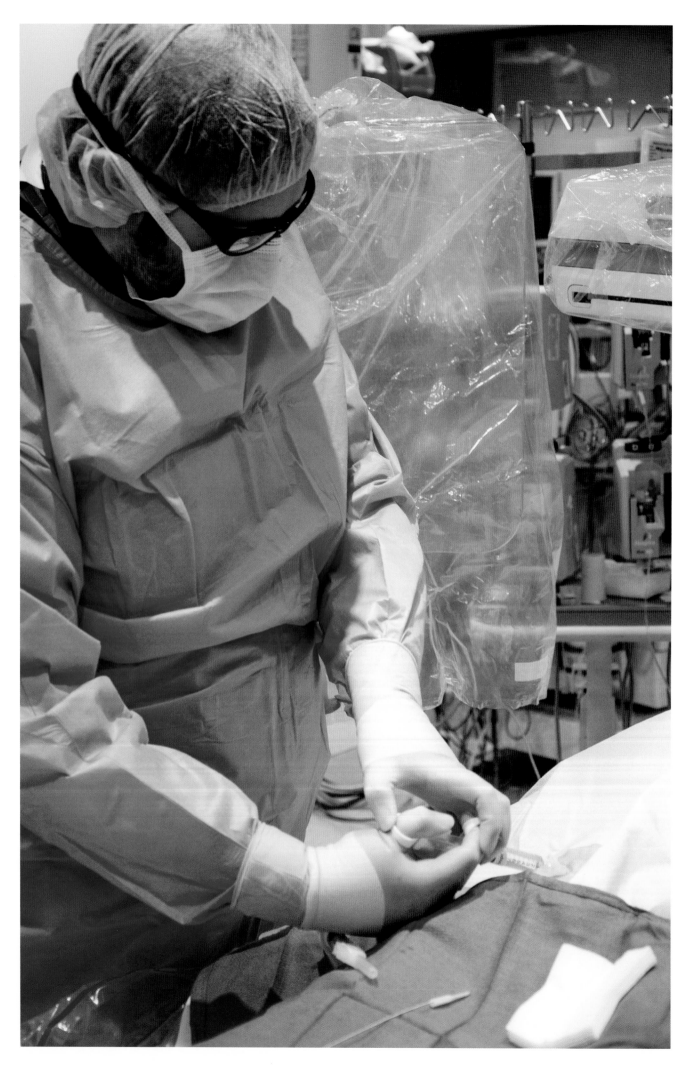

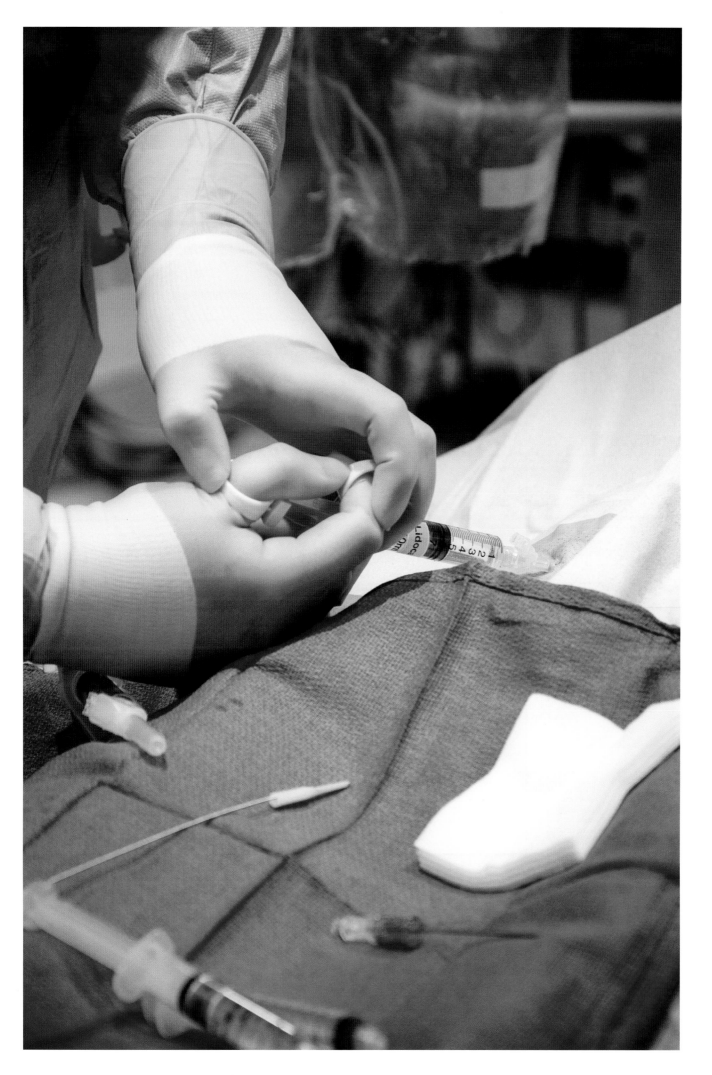

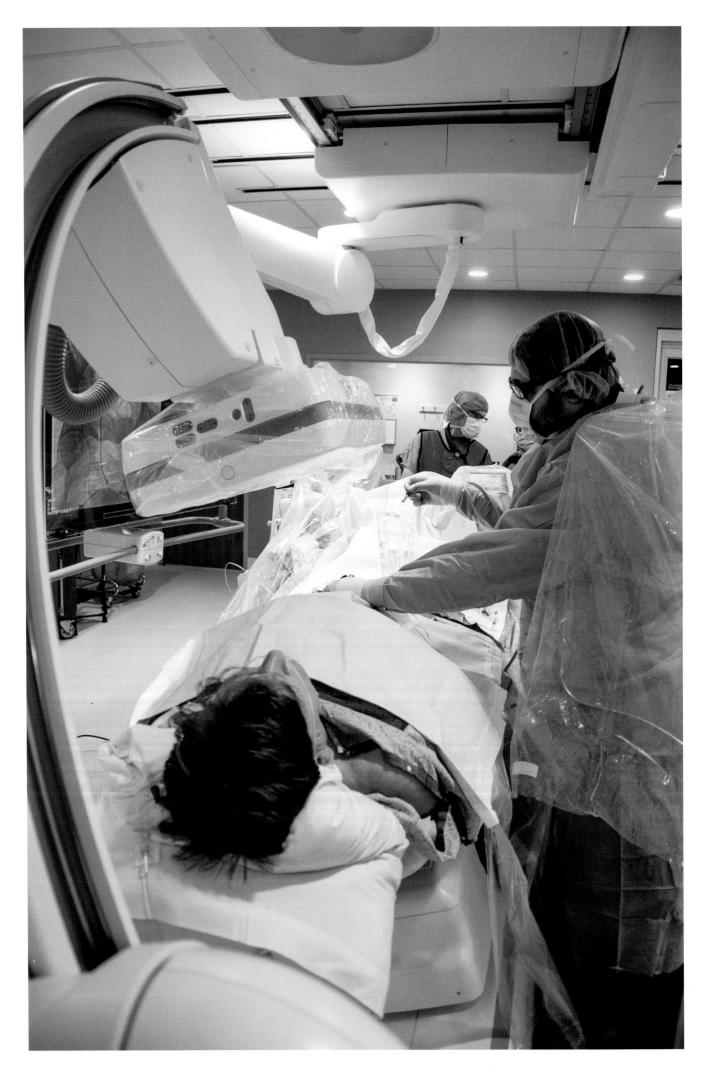

STERN CARDIOVASCULAR FOUNDATION

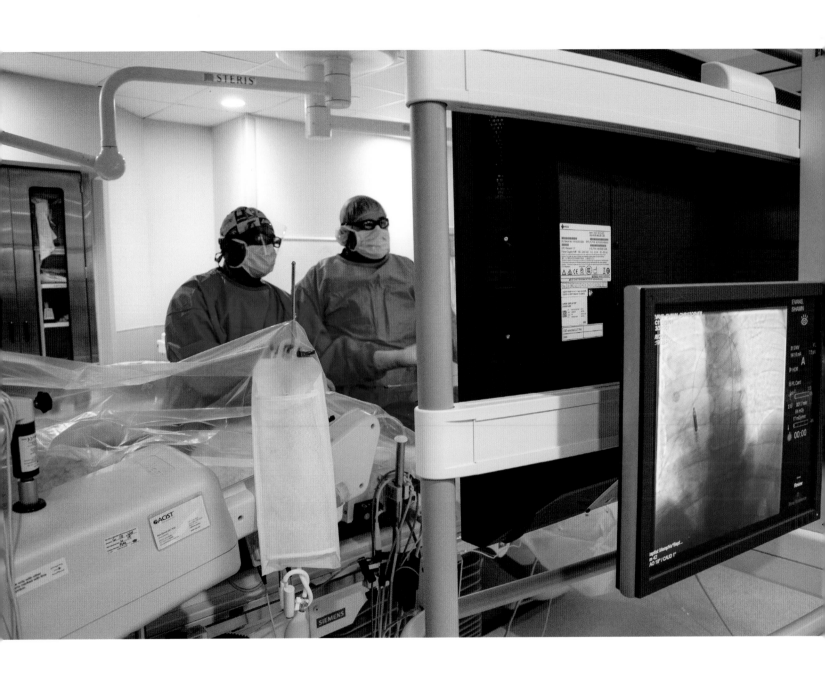

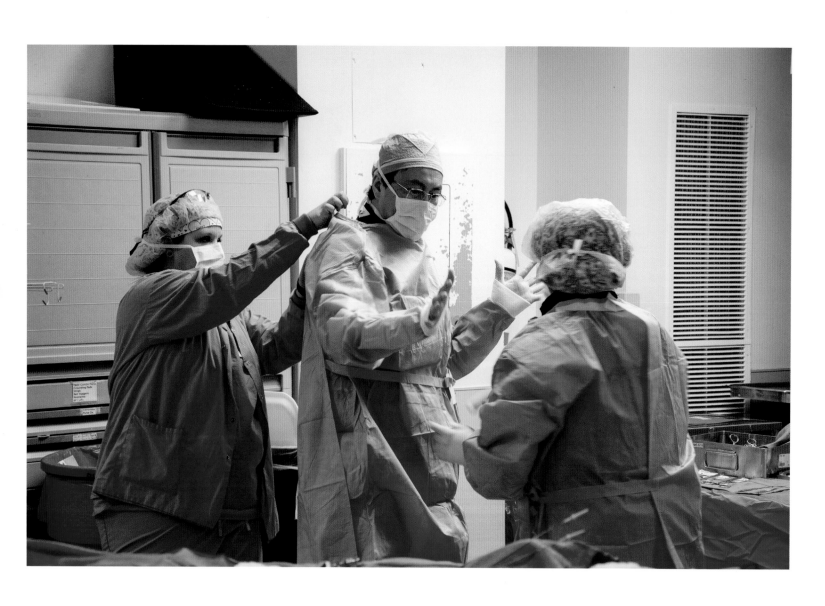

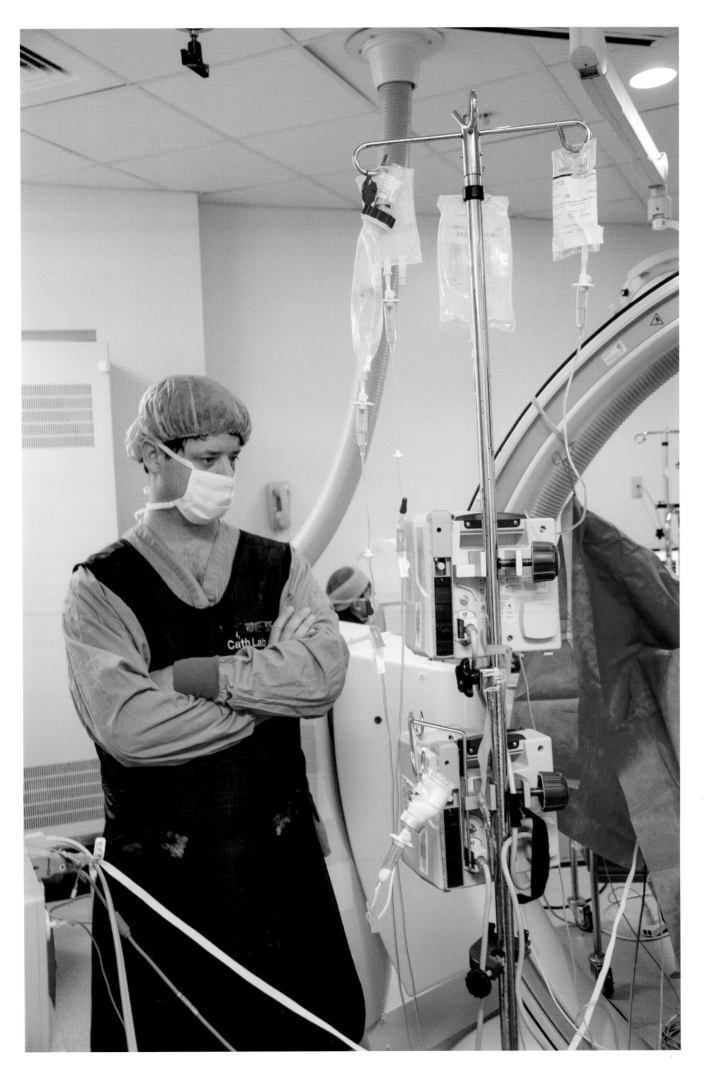

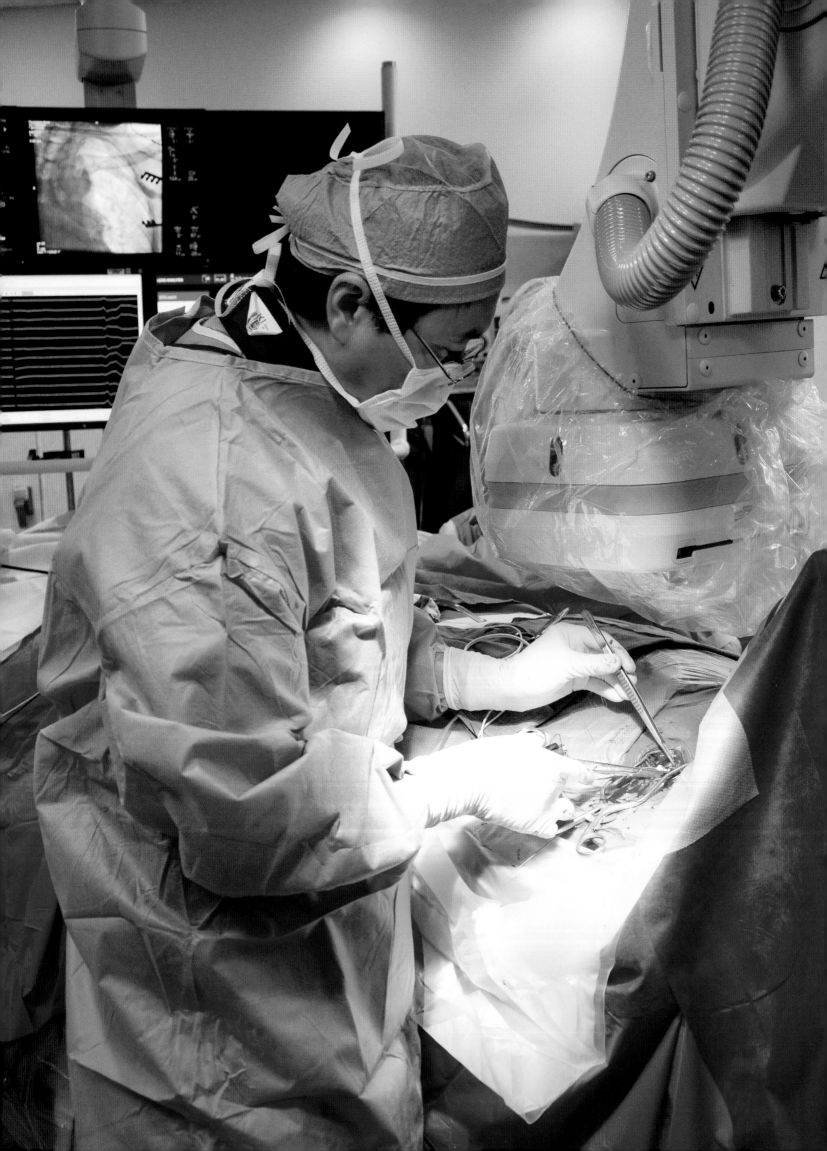

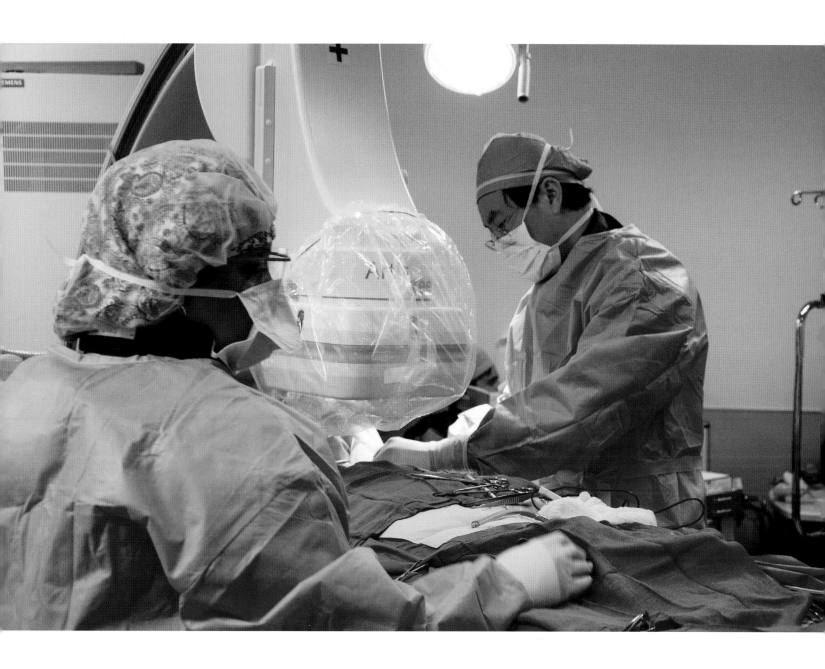

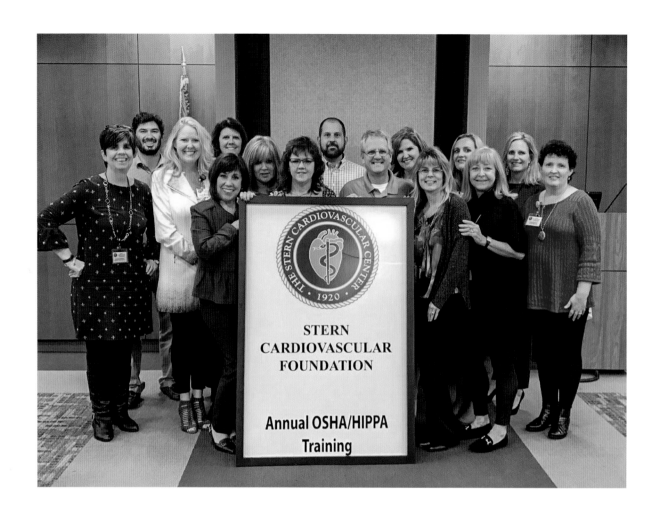

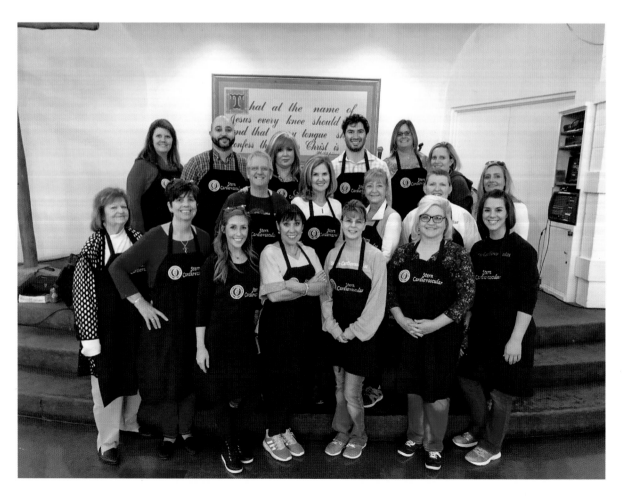

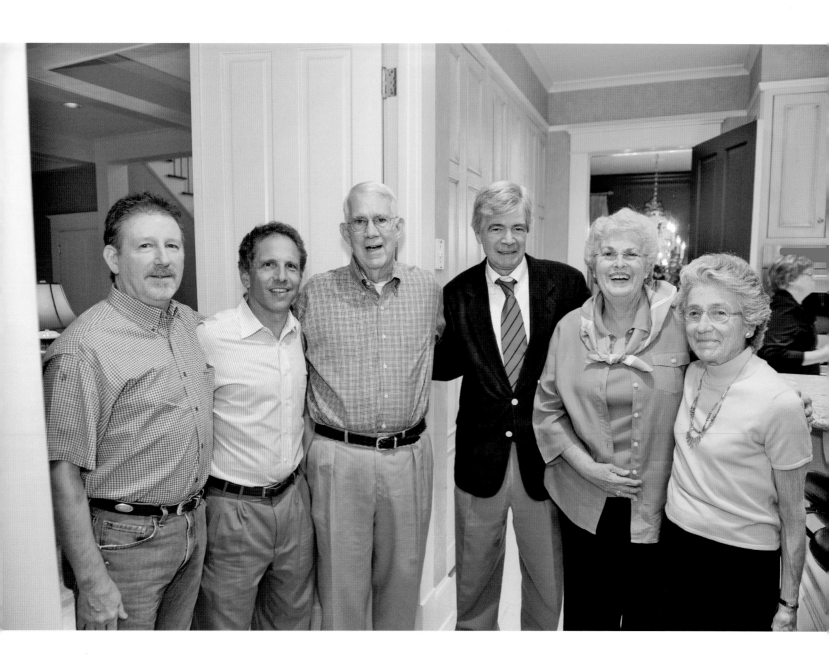

▲ Danny Eddlestone, Steven Gubin, David Holloway, Jan Turner, Lynn Holloway and Harriet Stern

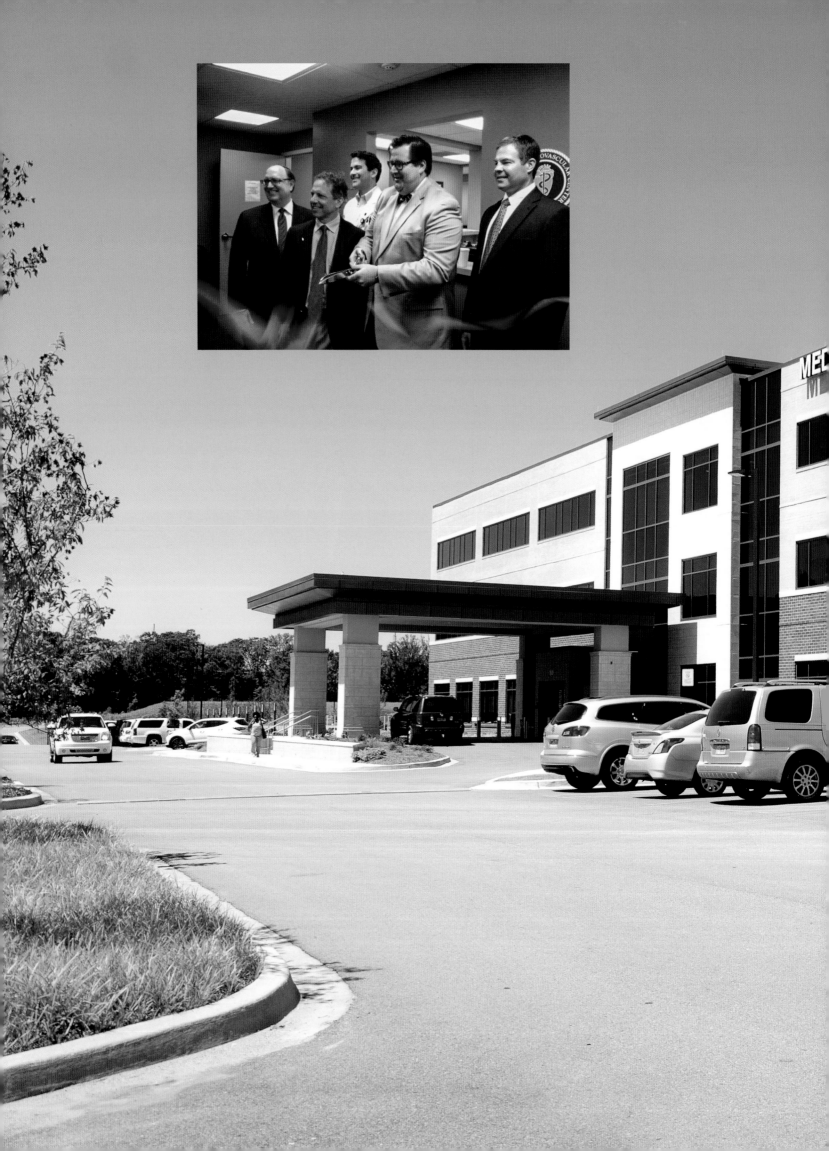

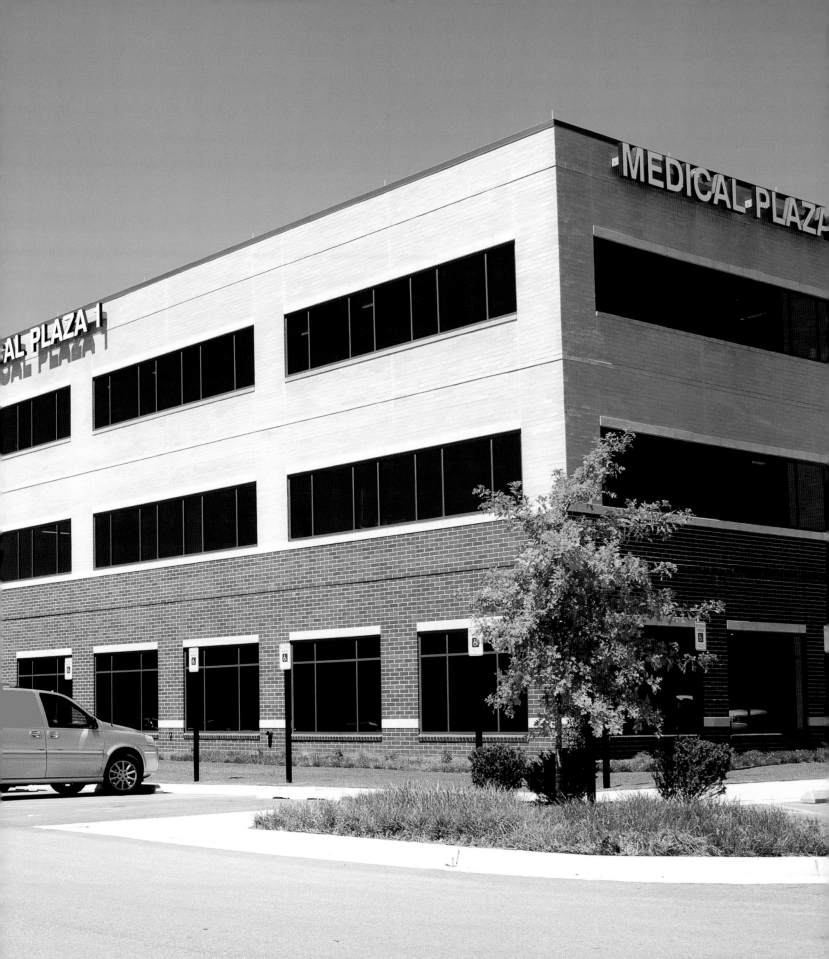

▲ The Stern Cardio Oxford Campus, and ribbon cutting at top left
photo by Stephanie Norwood

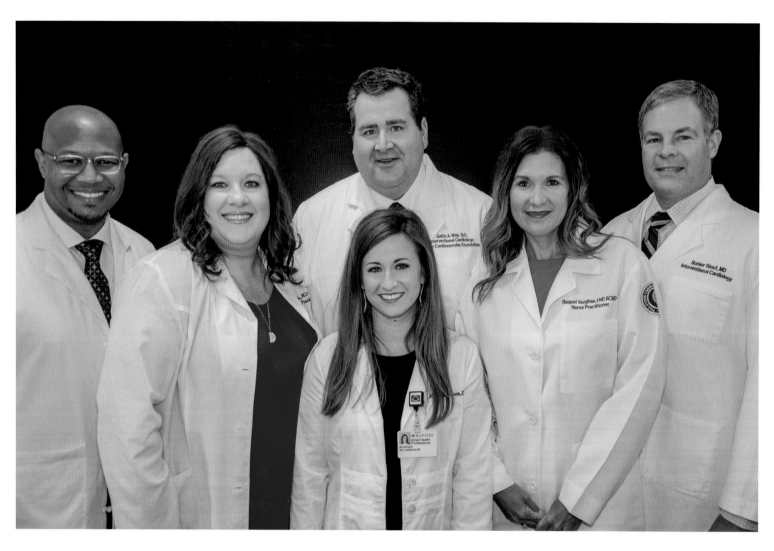

▲ The Stern Cardio Oxford staff and offices
photo by Stephanie Norwood

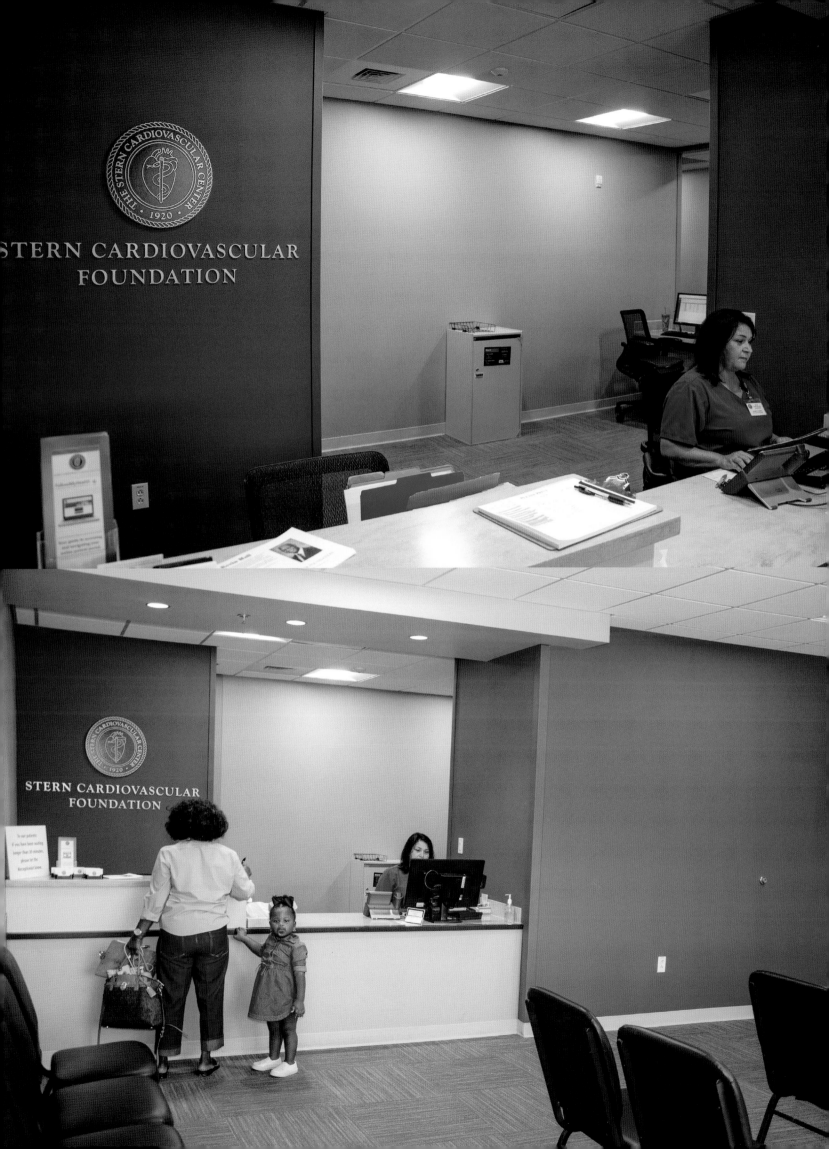

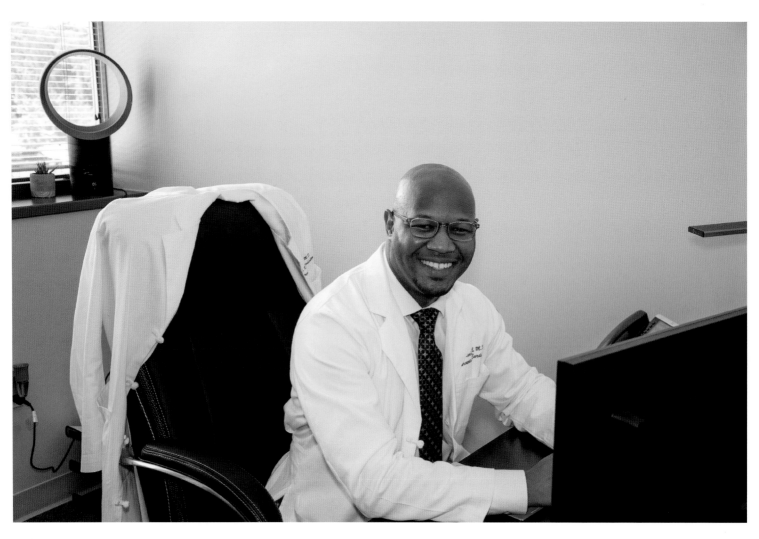

▲ Dr. James Kevin Hall

Photo by Stephanie Norwood

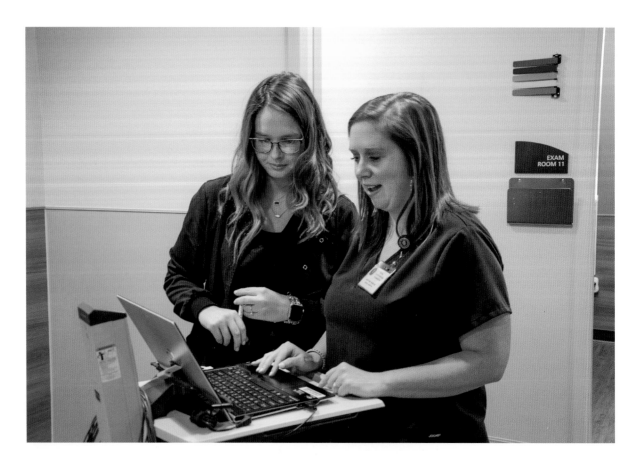

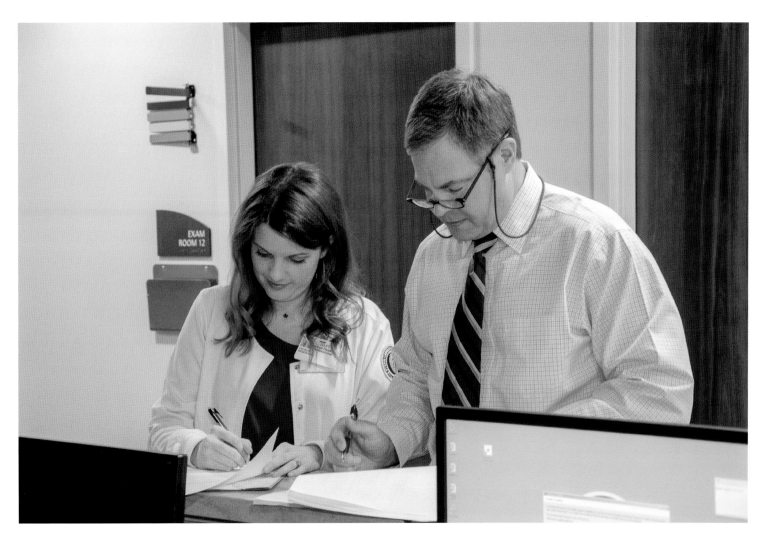

▲ Dr. J. Bunker Stout
Photo by Stephanie Norwood

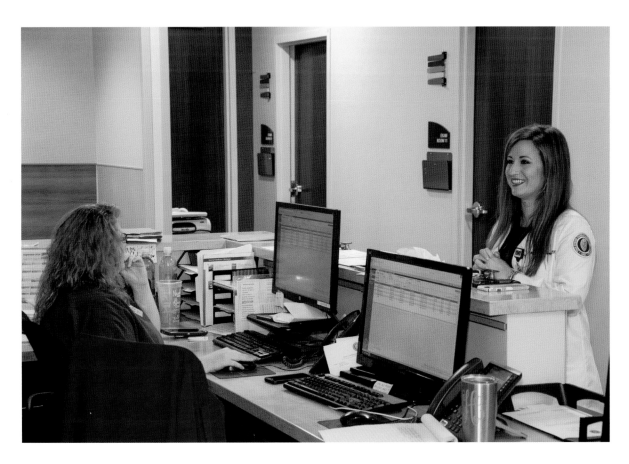

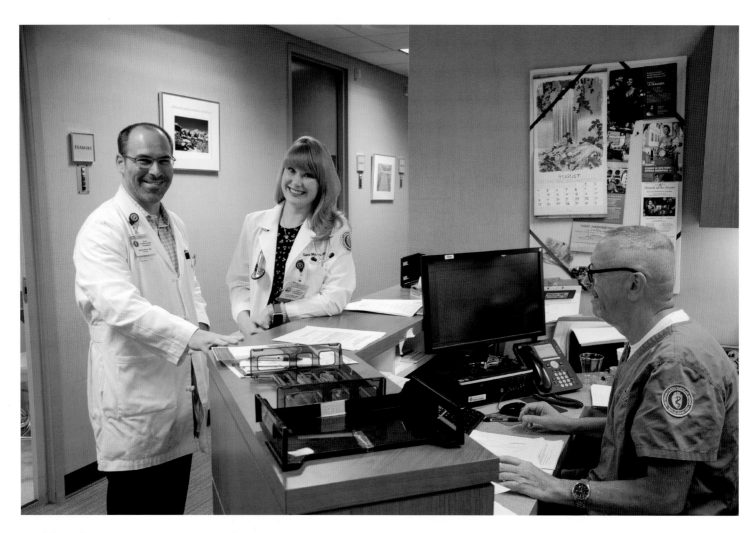

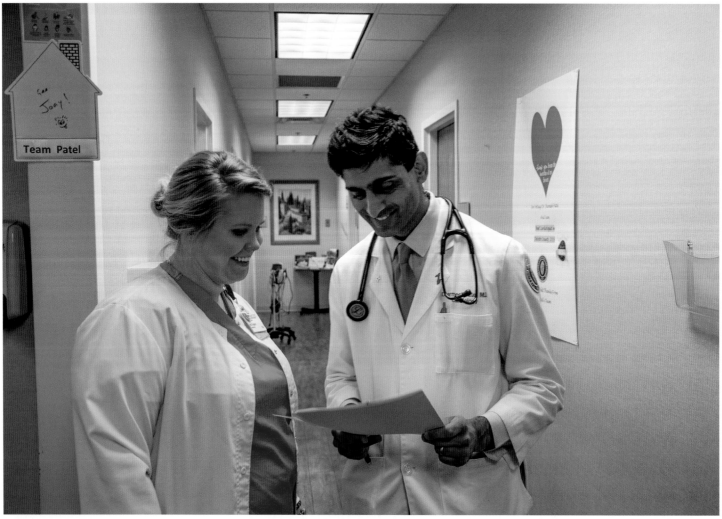

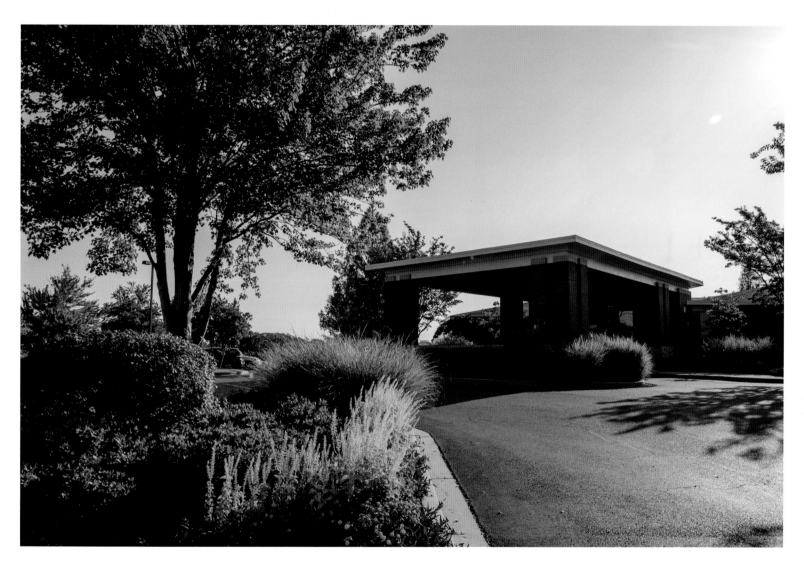

▲ Stern Cadiovascular Center in Southhaven
Photo by Stephanie Norwood

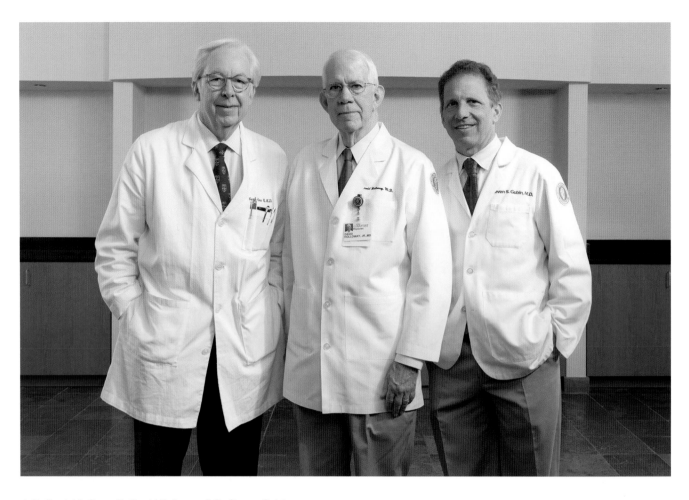

▲ Dr. Frank McGrew, Dr. David Holloway, & Dr. Steven Gubin

Photo credit: Stern Cardio

▼ Randy Meeks, Steven Gubin, & Sharon Goldstein

Photo by Stephanie Norwood

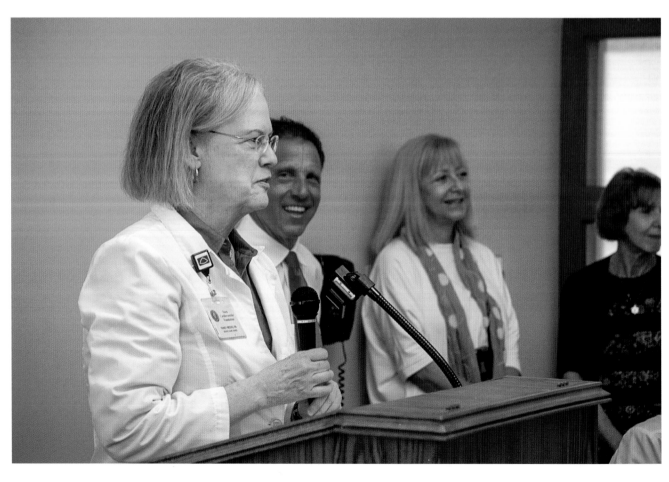

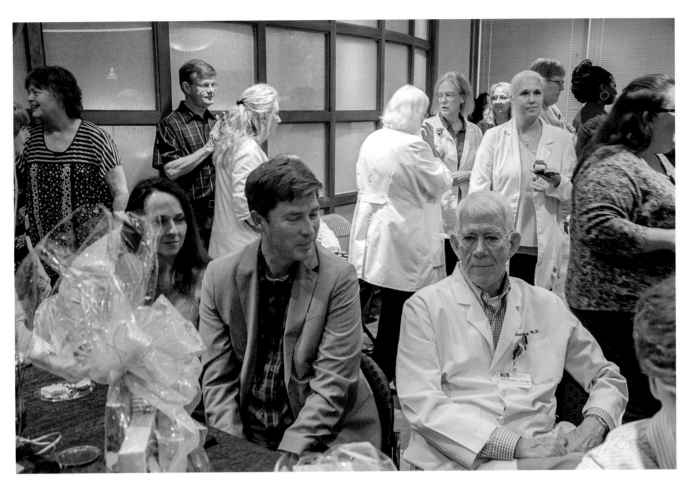

▲▼ Stern Party, Dr. Holloway (seated above), and Dr. Russo (seated below)

Photo photos by Stephanie Norwood

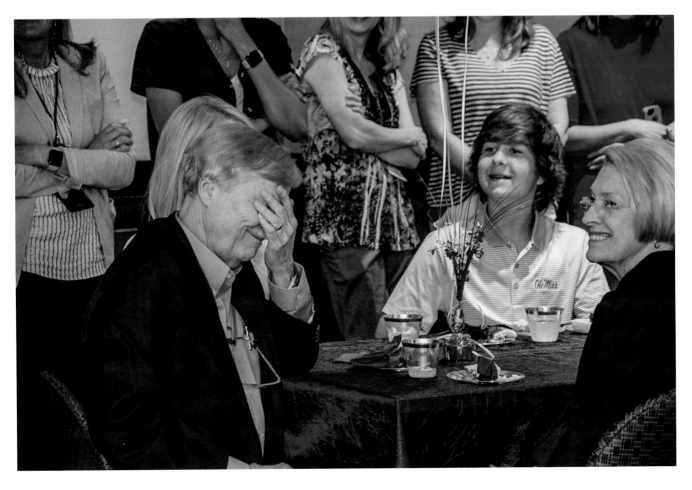

► Dr. Jiang Cui

Photo credit: Stern Cardio

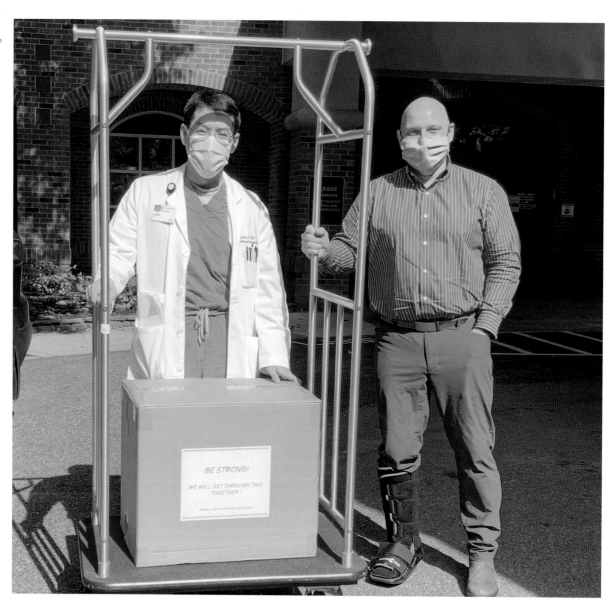

► Staff at the Wolf River location

Photo by Stephanie Norwood

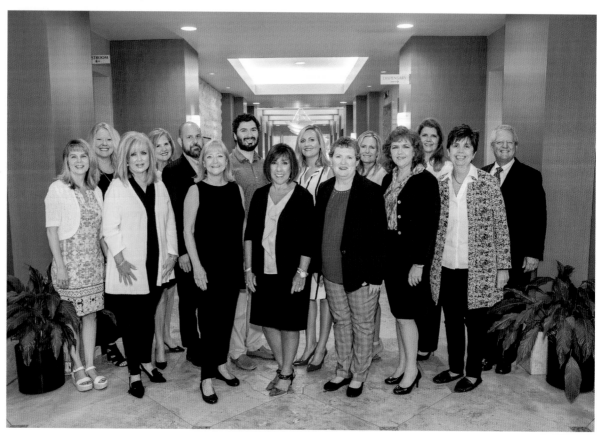

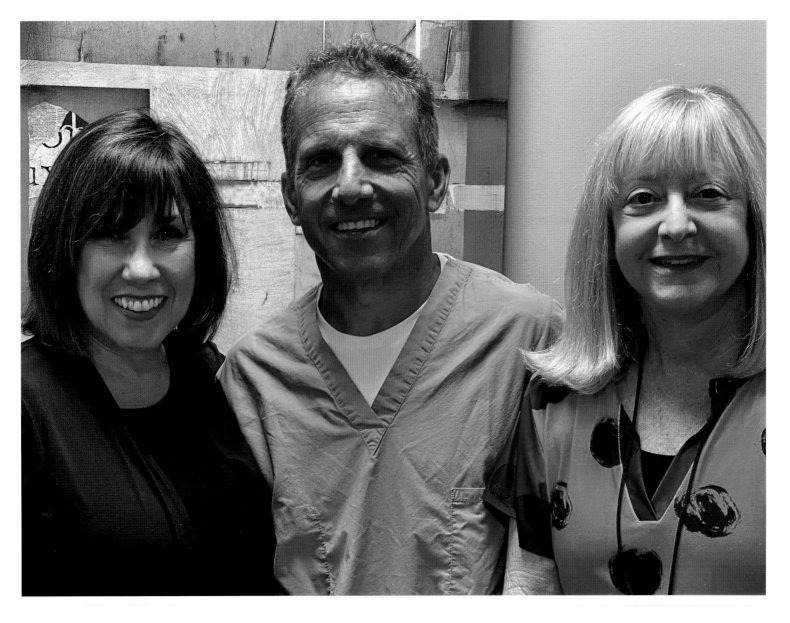

▲ Debbie Eddlestone,
Dr. Steven Gubin, and
Sharon Goldstein

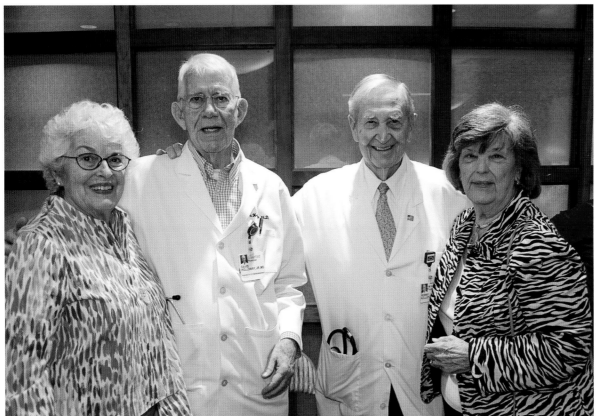

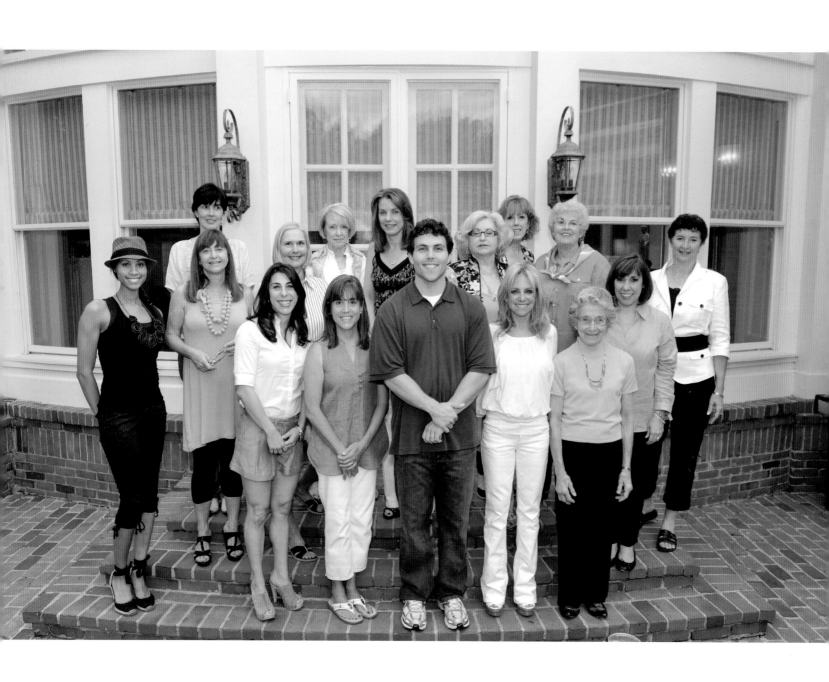

132   S<small>TERN</small> C<small>ARDIOVASCULAR</small> F<small>OUNDATION</small>

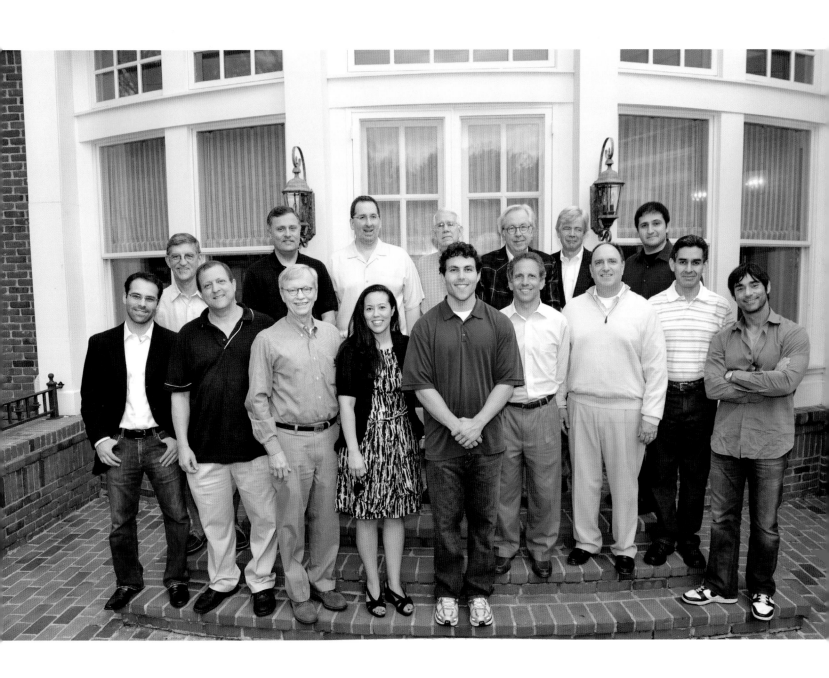

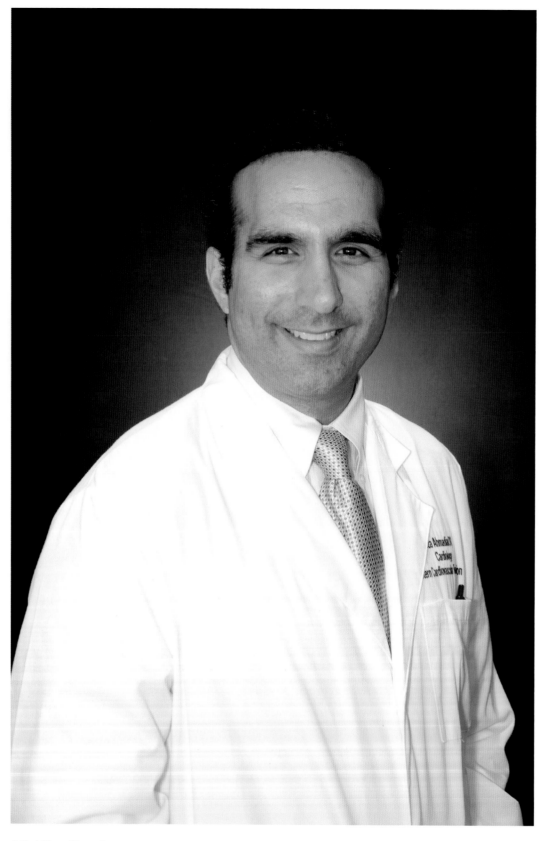

▲ Dr. H Reza Ahmadian

Photo by Stephanie Norwood

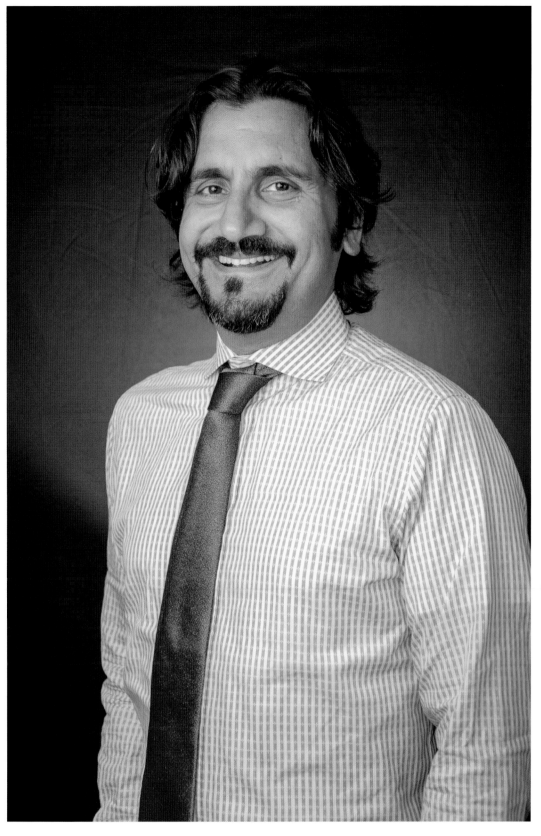

▲ Dr. Yaser Cheema

Photo by Stephanie Norwood

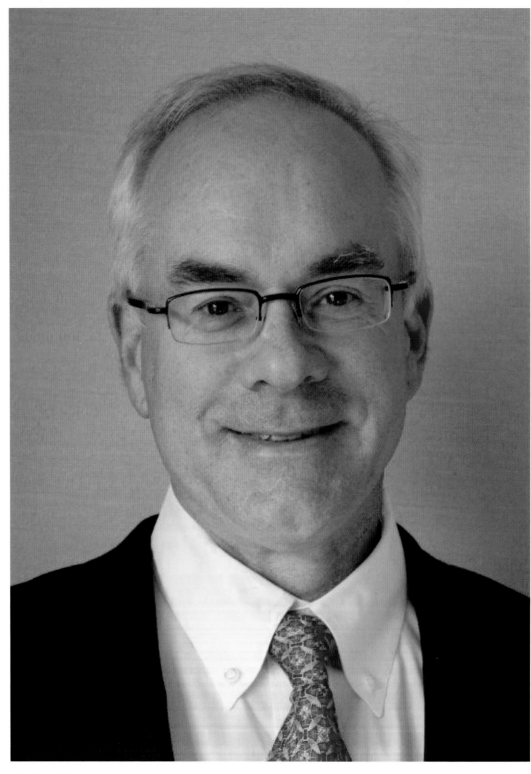

▲ Dr. Ray Allen

Photo credit Stern Cardiovascular Foundation

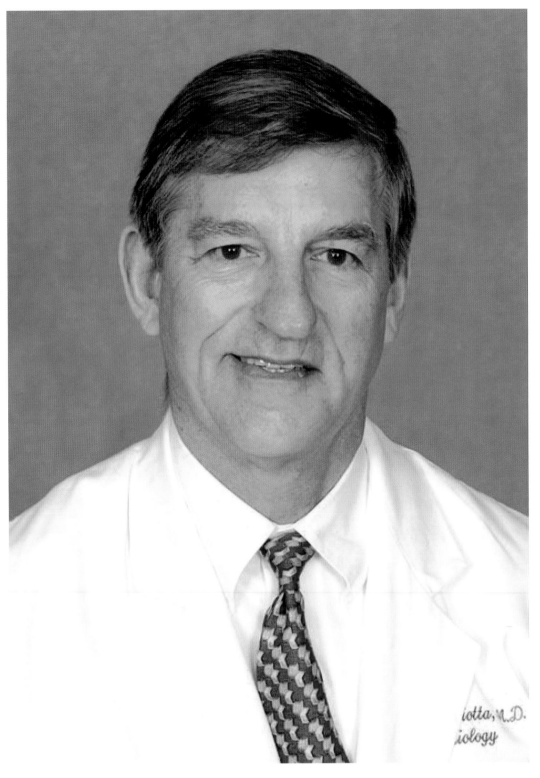

▲ Dr. Larry Spiotta

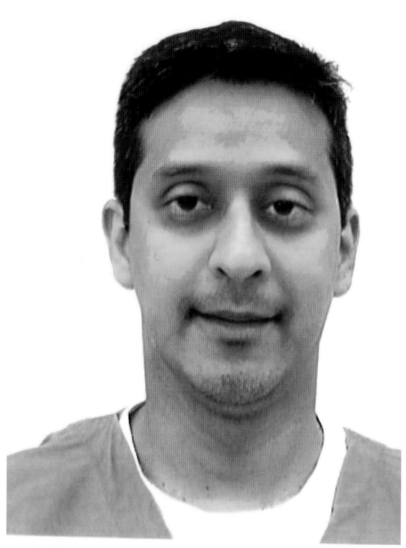

▲ Dr. Haris Zafarullah

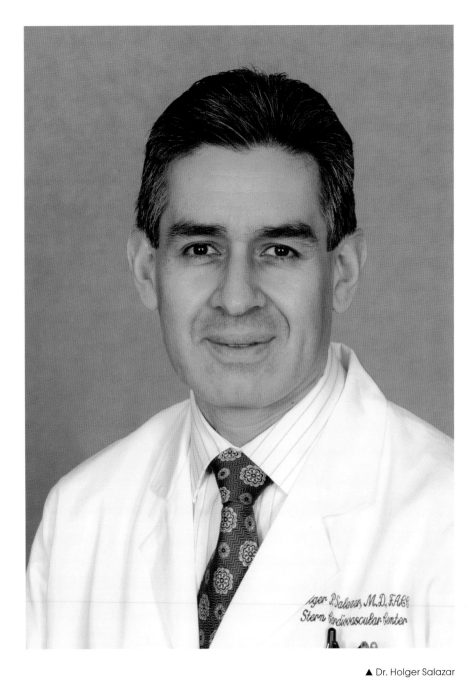

▲ Dr. Holger Salazar

Photo credit Stern Cardiovascular
Foundation

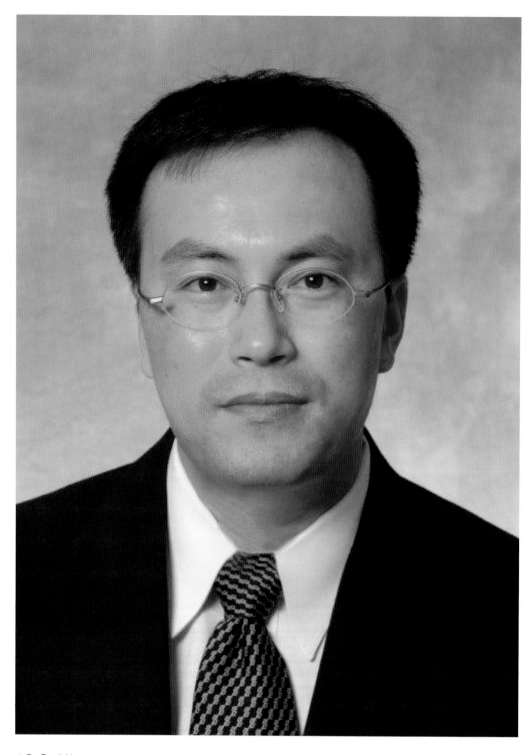

▲ Dr. David Lan

Photo credit Stern Cardiovascular
Foundation

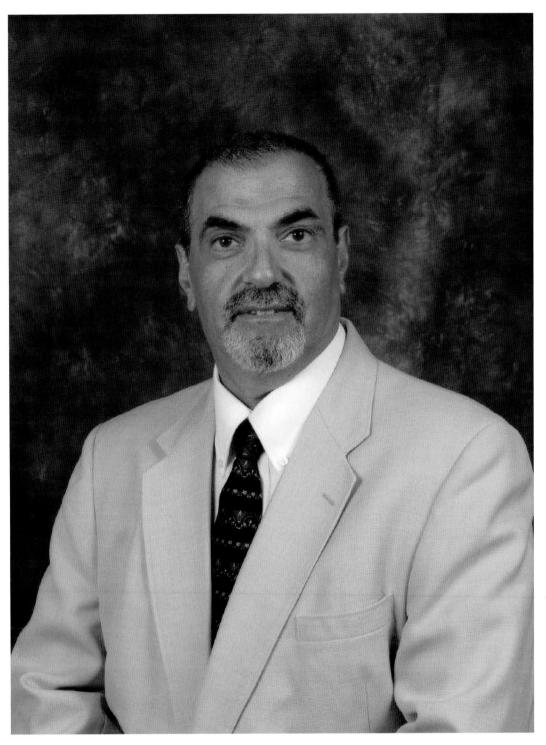

▲ Dr. Louis Caruso
Photo credit: Stern Cardiovascular Foundation

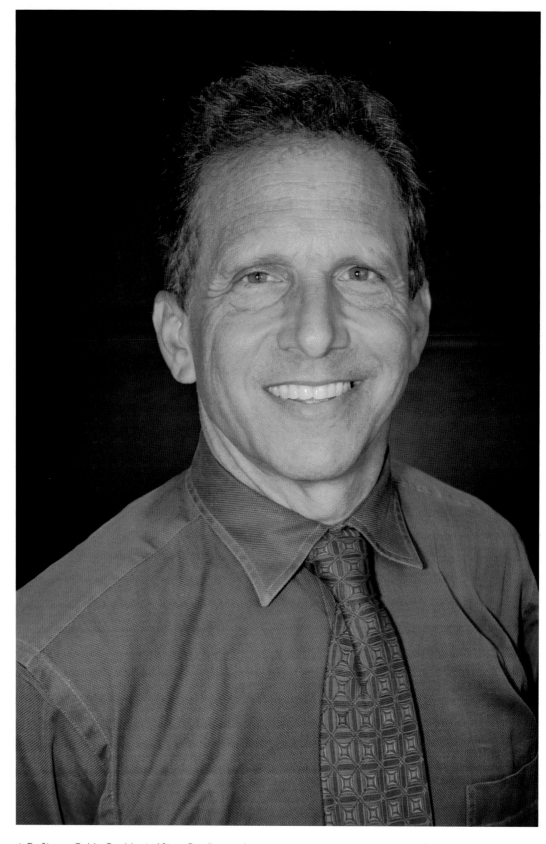

▲ Dr. Steven Gubin, President of Stern Cardiovascular

Photo by Stephanie Norwood

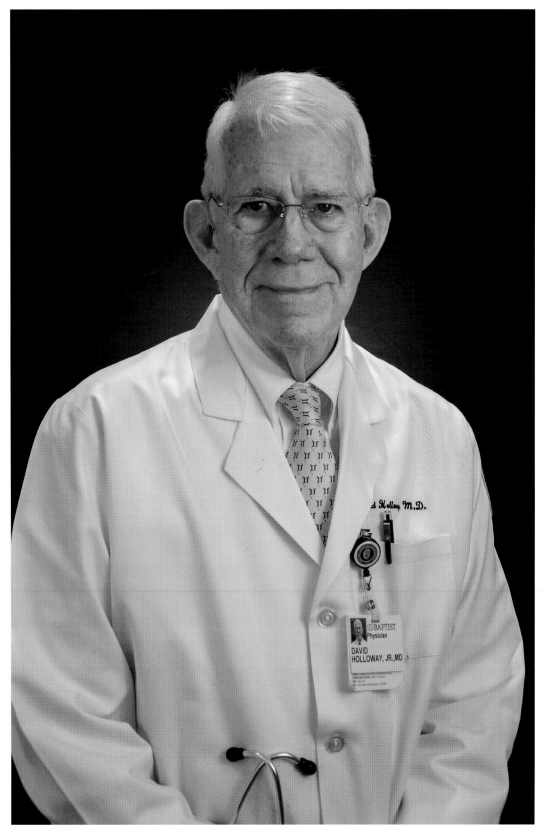

▲ Dr. David Holloway, Jr.
Photo by Stephanie Norwood

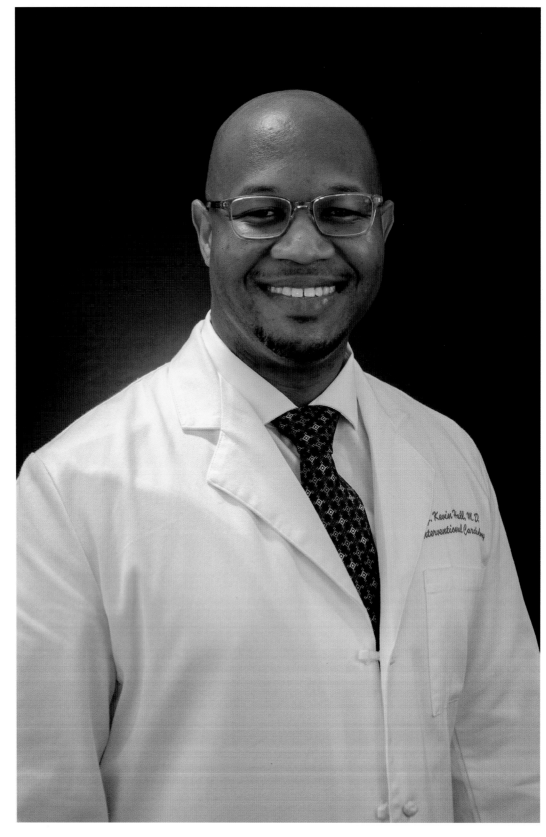

▲ Dr. James Kevin Hall

Photo by Stephanie Norwood

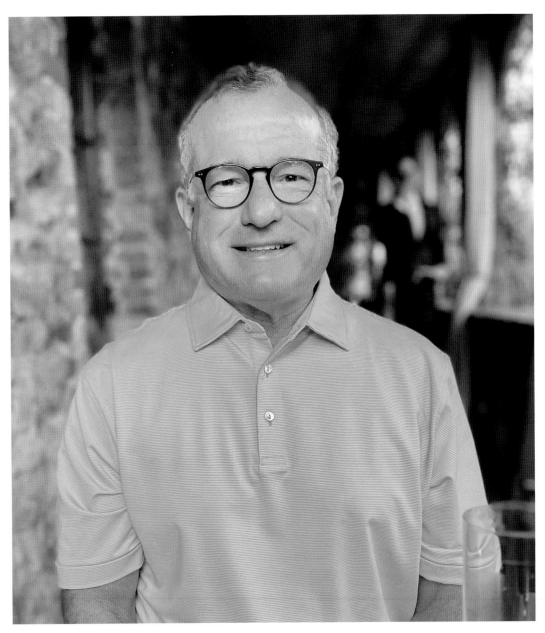

▲ Dr David Wolford
Photo by Stephanie Norwood

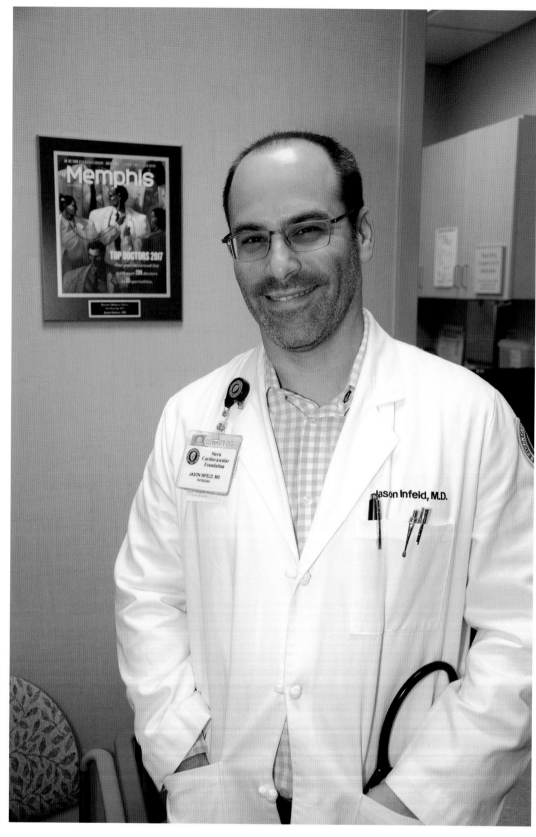

▲ Dr. Jason L Infeld

Photo by Stephanie Norwood

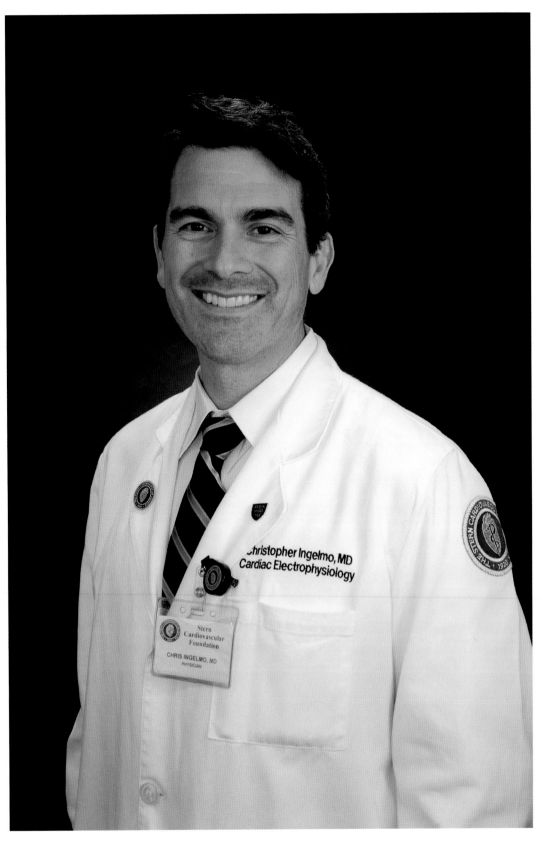

▲ Dr. Christopher p. Ingelmo
Photo by Stephanie Norwood

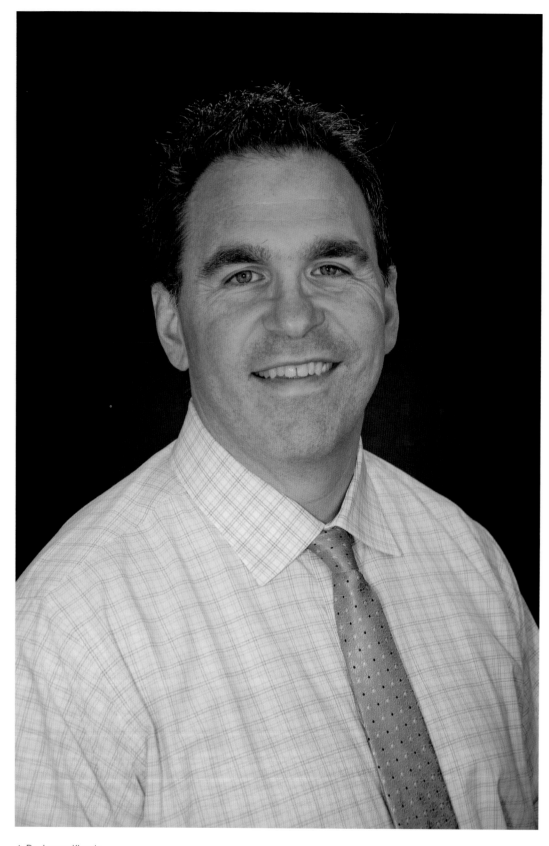

▲ Dr. James Klemis

Photo by Stephanie Norwood

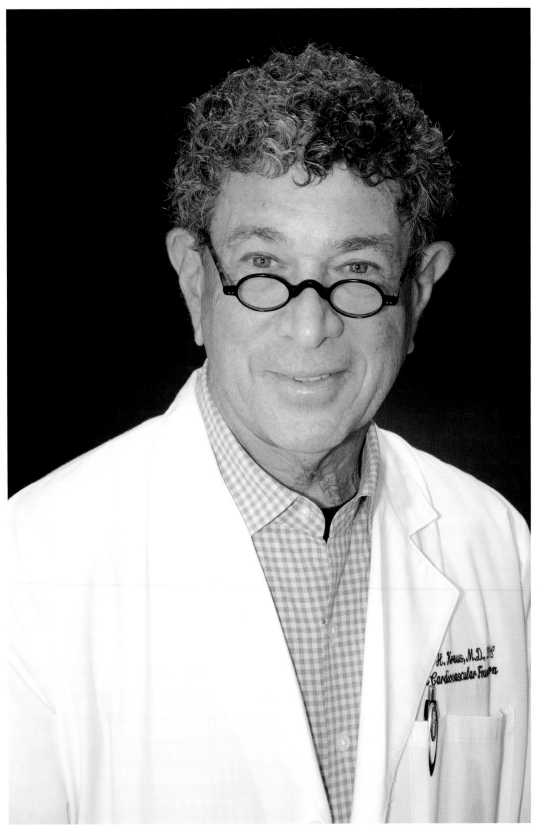

▲ Dr David H Kraus
Photo by Stephanie Norwood

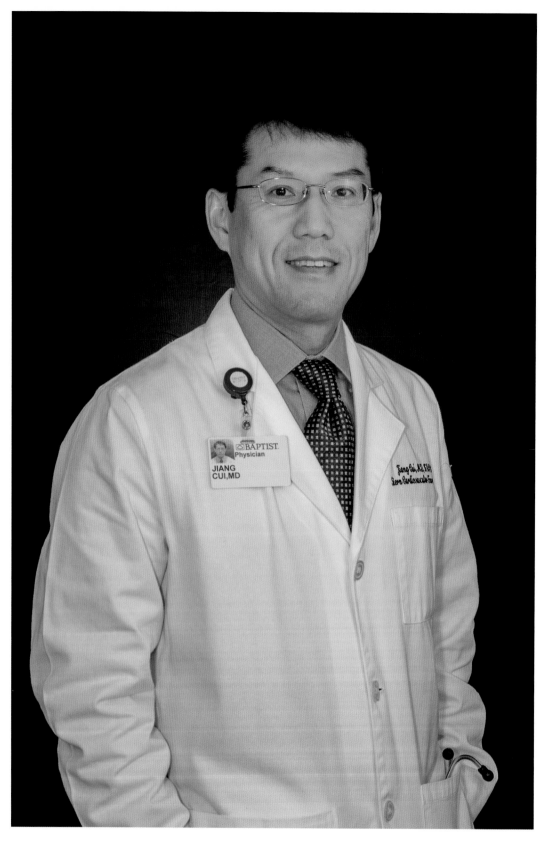

▲ Dr. Jiang Cui

Photo by Stephanie Norwood

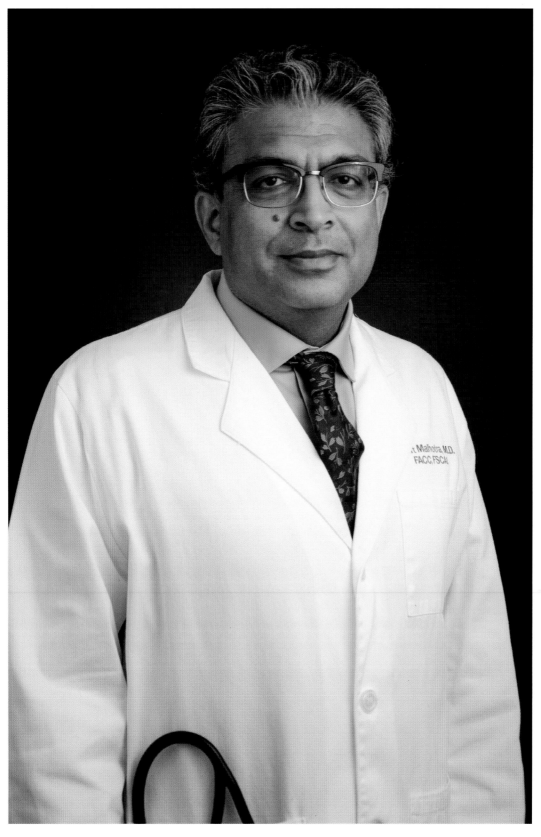

▲ Dr. Amit Malholtra
Photo by Stephanie Norwood

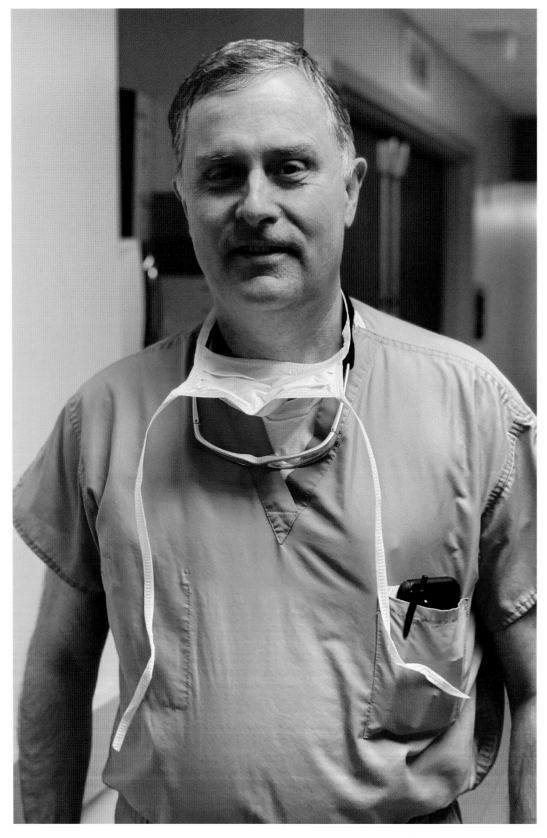

▲ Dr Mark Coppess

Photo by Stephanie Norwood

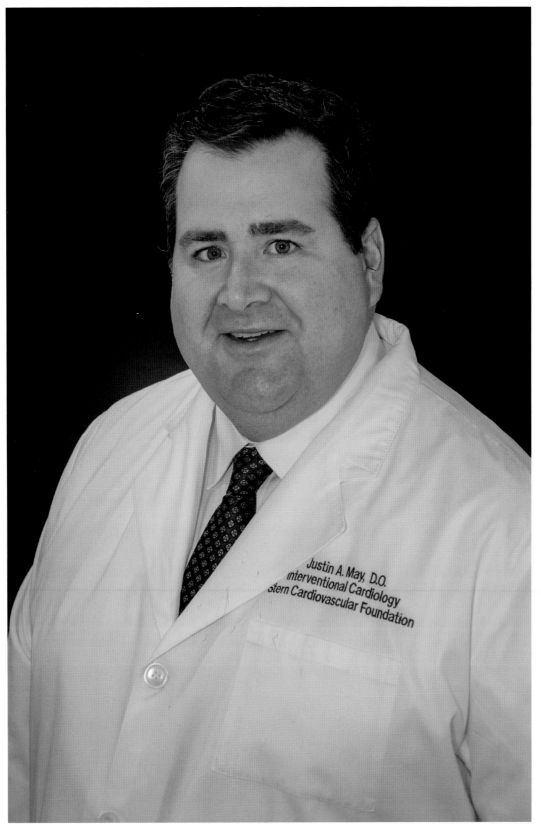

▲ Dr. Justin A. May
Photo by Stephanie Norwood

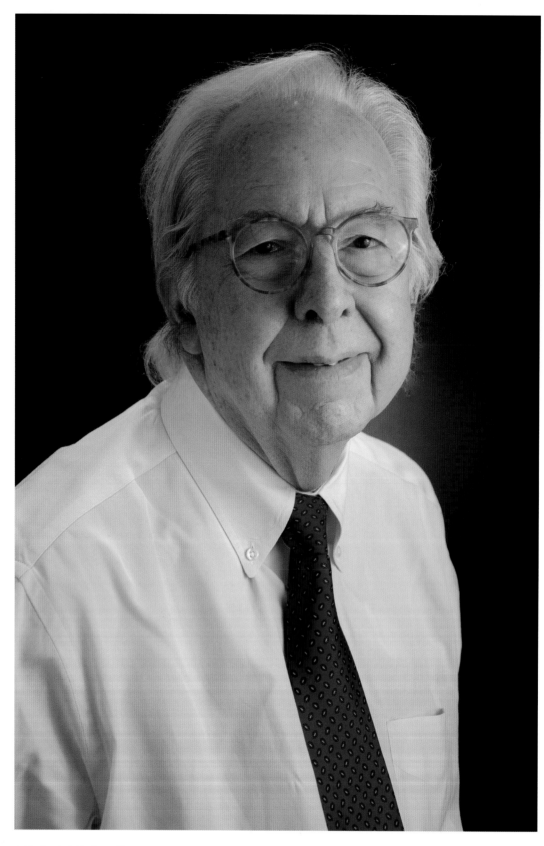

▲ Dr. Frank A McGrew III

Photo by Stephanie Norwood

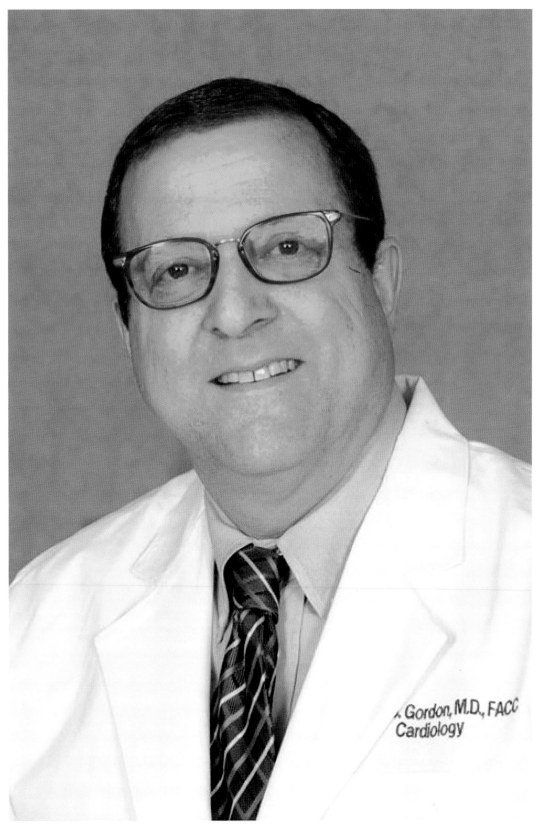

▲ Dr. Richard Gordon
Photo credit Stern Cardiovascular Foundation

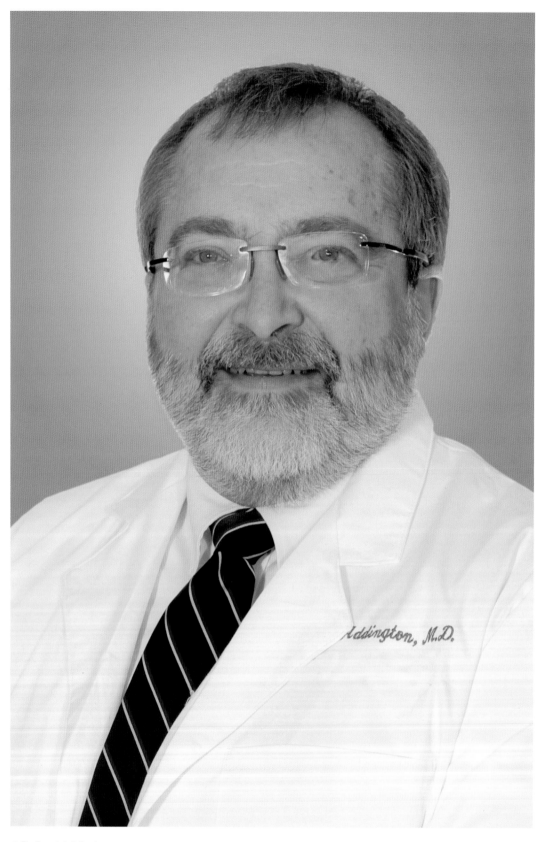

▲ Dr. Brent Addington

Photo by Stephanie Norwood

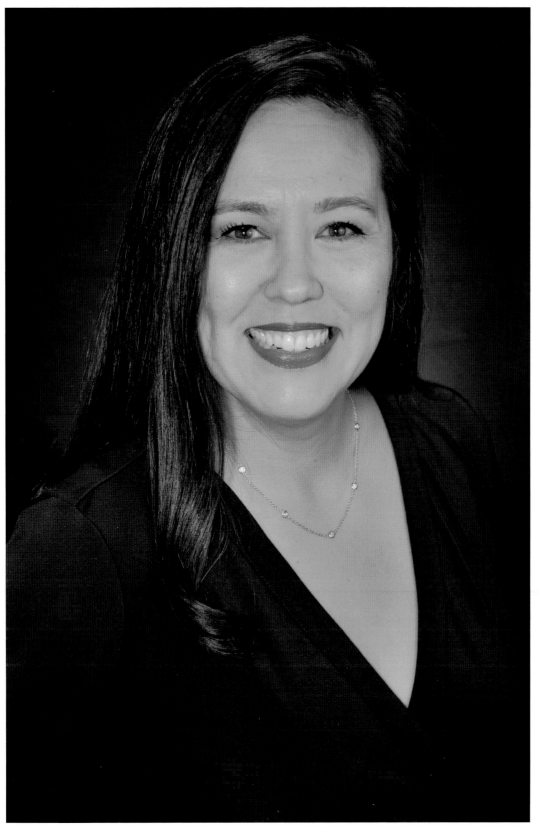

▲ Dr. Jennifer S Morrow
Photo by Stephanie Norwood

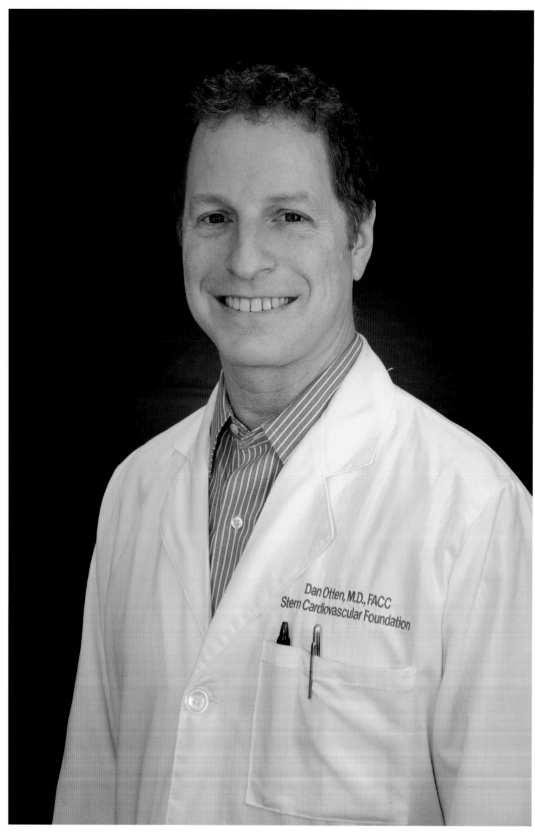

▲ Dr. Daniel E. Otten

Photo by Stephanie Norwood

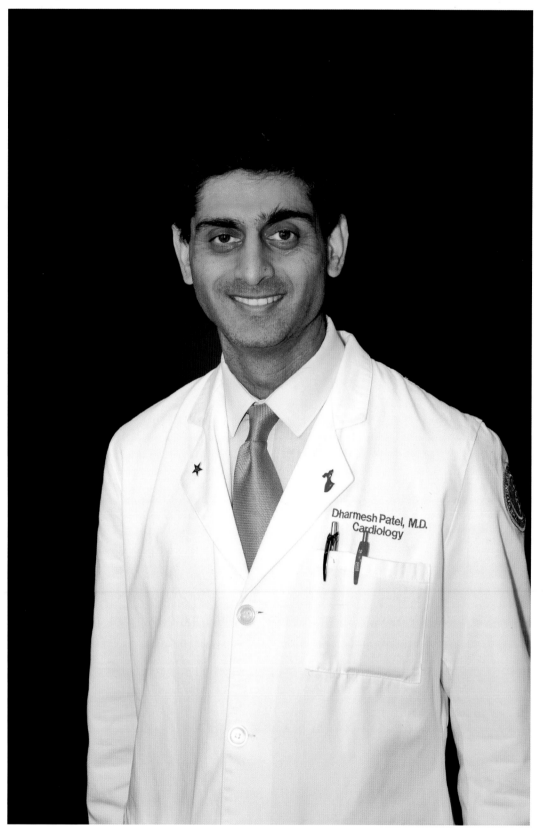

▲ Dr. Dharmesh S. Patel
Photo by Stephanie Norwood

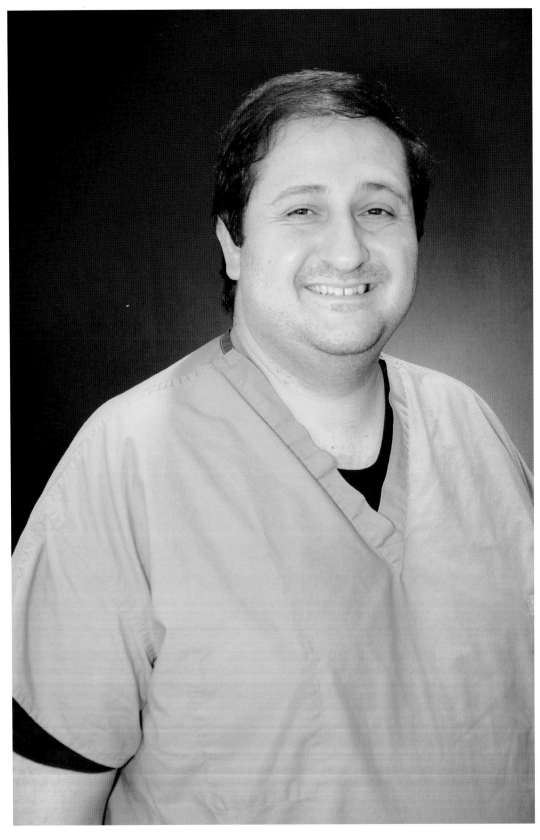

▲ Dr. Basil M. Paulus

Photo by Stephanie Norwood

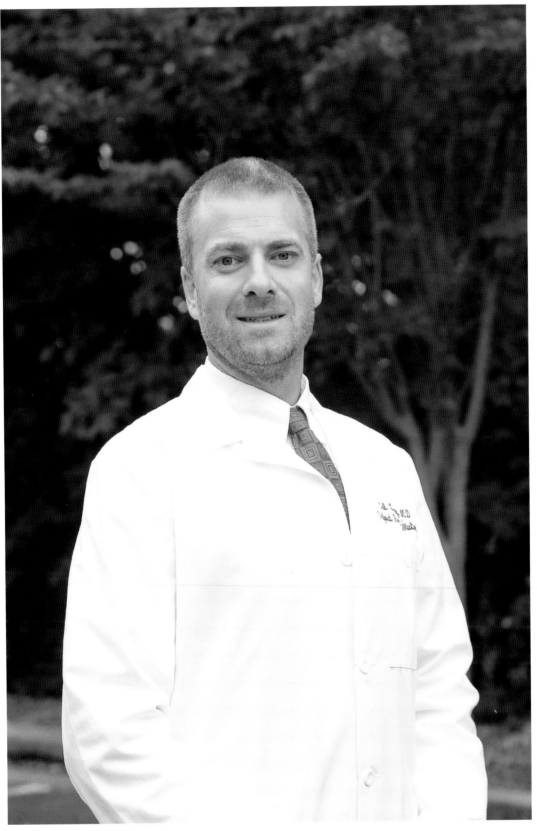

▲ Dr. Charles A. Laney
Photo by Stephanie Norwood

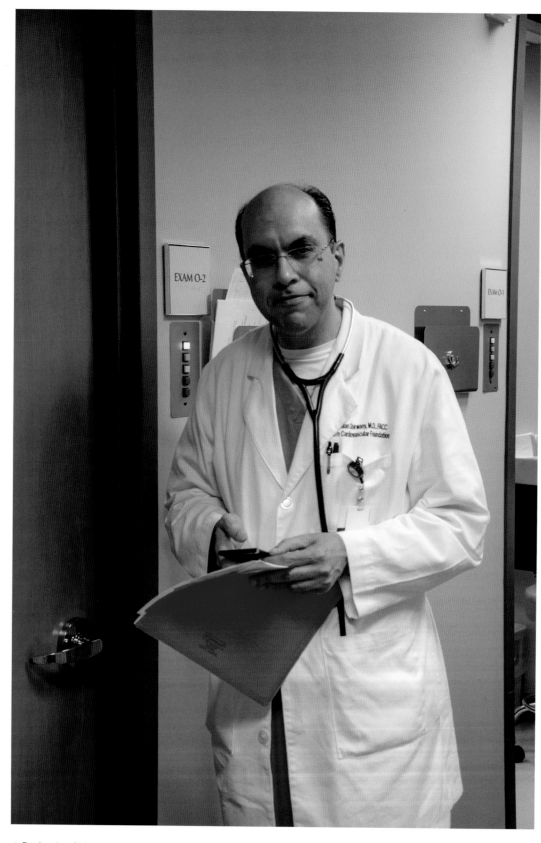

▲ Dr. Arsalan Shirwany

Photo by Stephanie Norwood

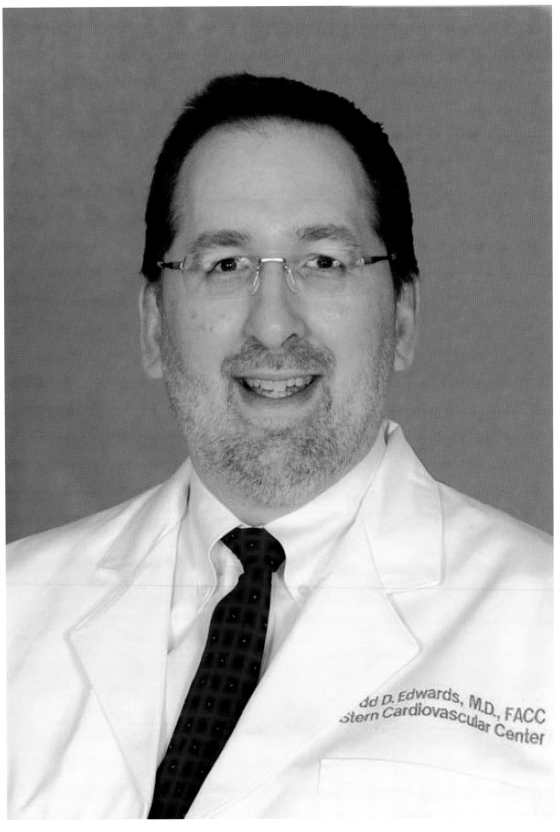

▲ Dr. Todd Edwards
Photo credit Stern Cardiovascular Foundation

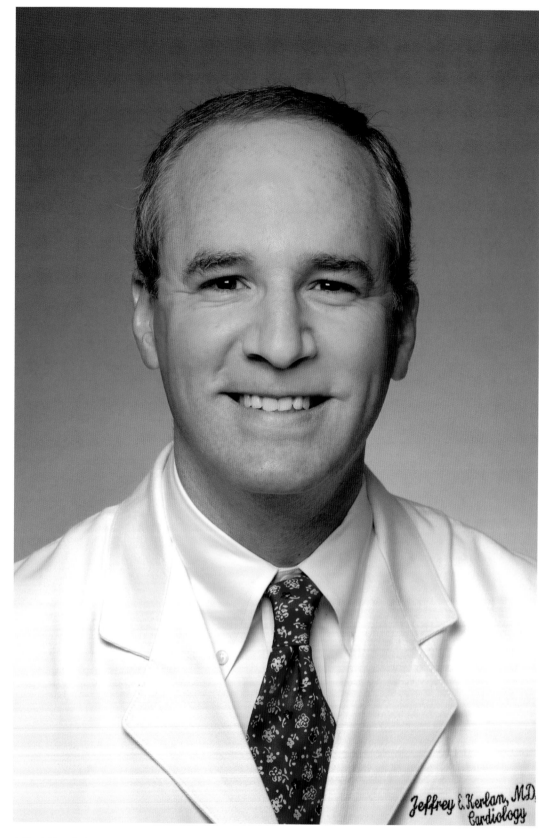

▲ Dr. Jeffrey Kerlan

Photo by Stephanie Norwood

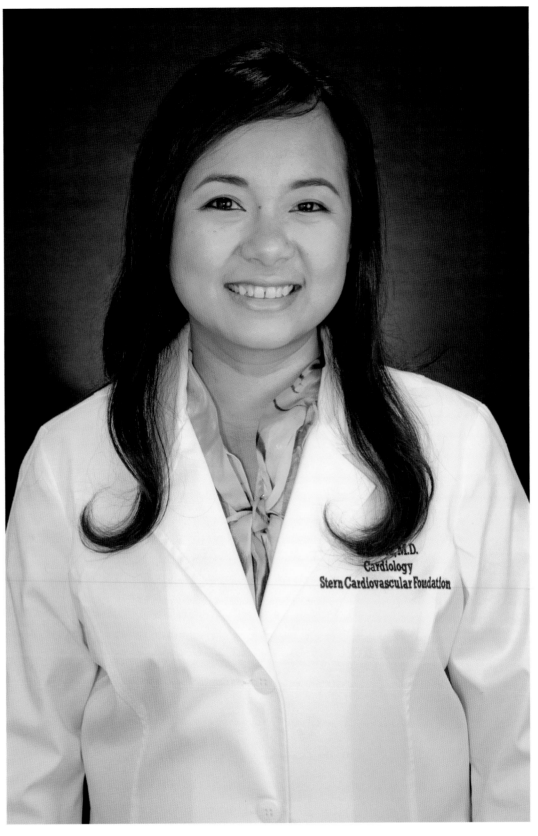

▲ Dr. Ei K Swe
Photo by Stephanie Norwood

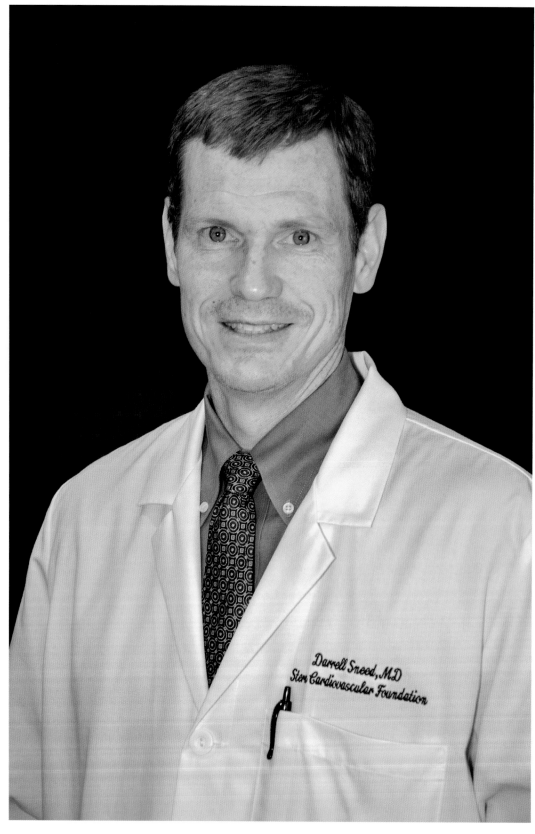

▲ Dr. Darrell Sneed

Photo by Stephanie Norwood

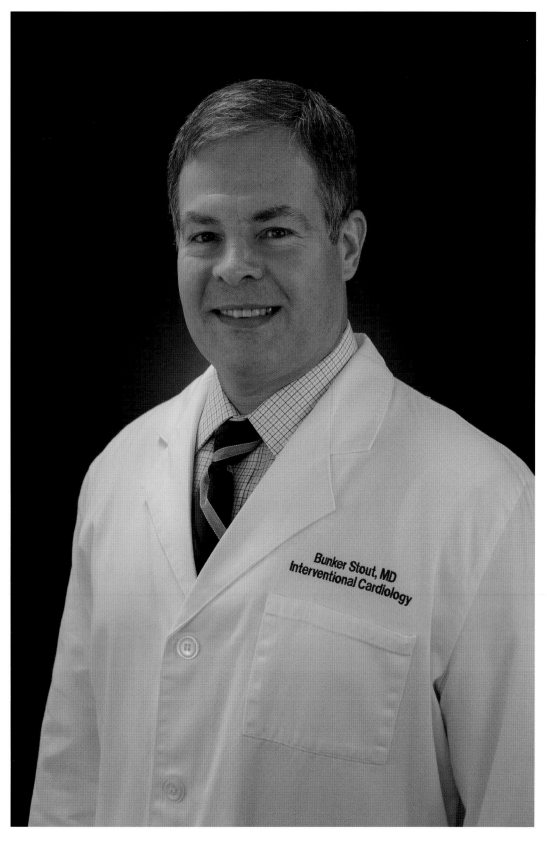

▲ Dr. J. Bunker Stout
Photo by Stephanie Norwood

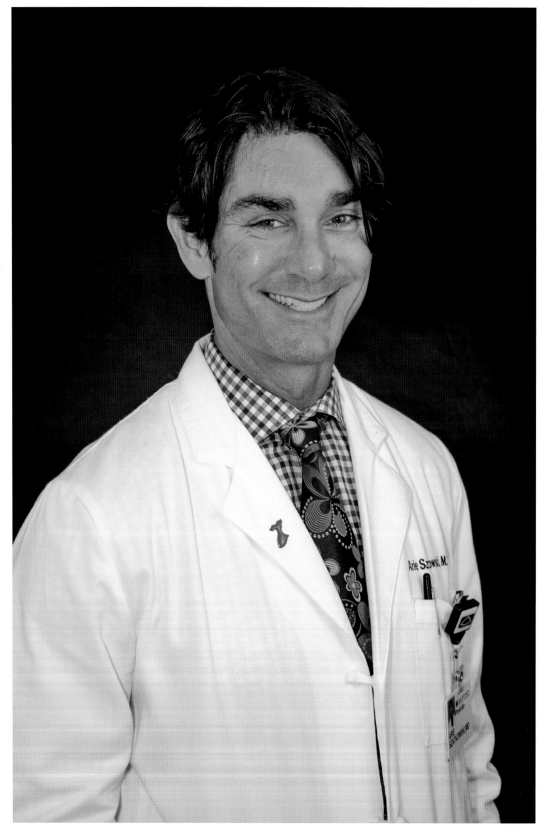

▲ Dr. Arie Szatkowski

Photo by Stephanie Norwood

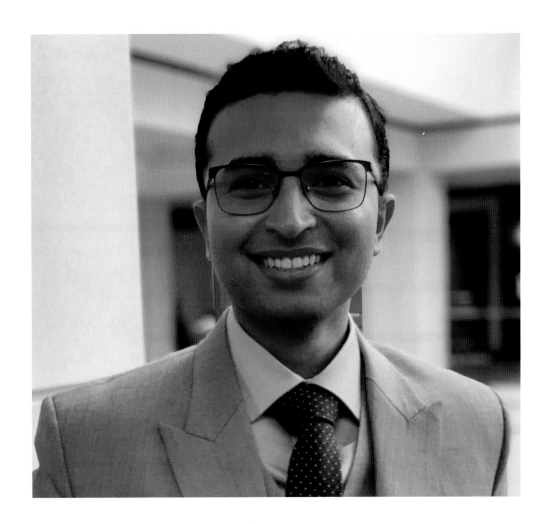

◀ Dr. Shankho Ganguli
Photo credit Stern Cardiovascular
Foundation

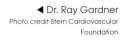

◀ Dr. Ray Gardner
Photo credit Stern Cardiovascular
Foundation

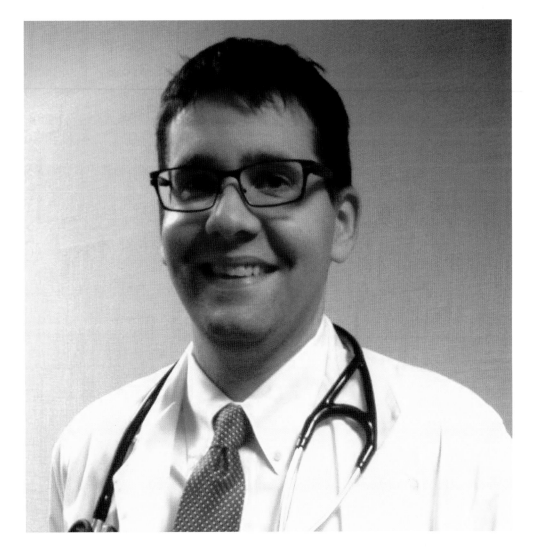

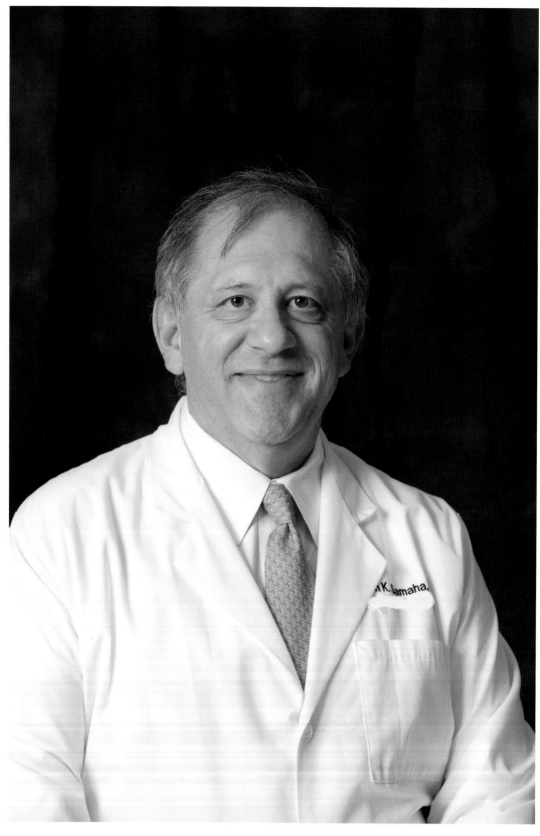

▲ Dr. Joseph Samaha

Photo by Stephanie Norwood

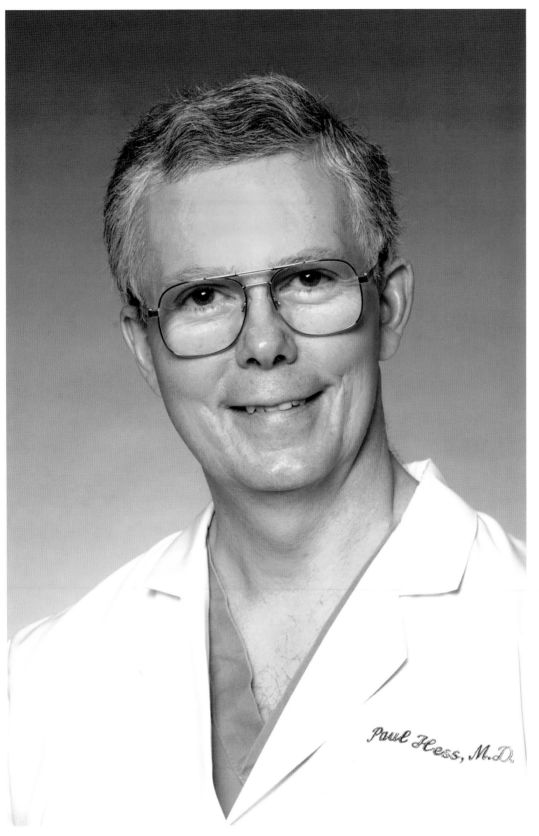

▲ Dr. Paul Hess
Photo credit Stern Cardiovascular Foundation

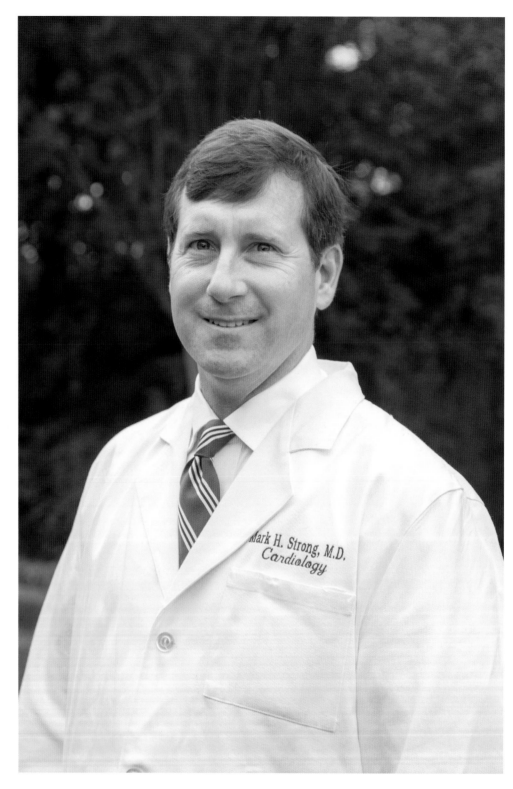

▲ Dr. Mark H. Strong
Photo by Stephanie Norwood

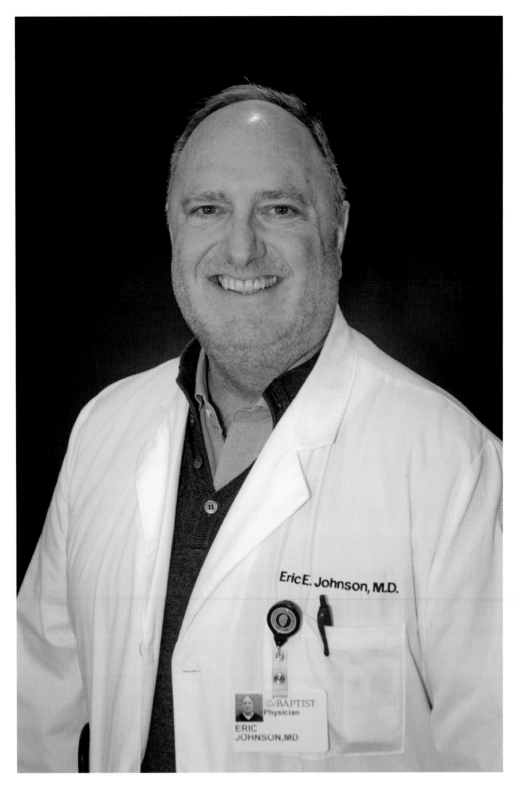

▲ Dr. Eric Johnson
Photo by Stephanie Norwood

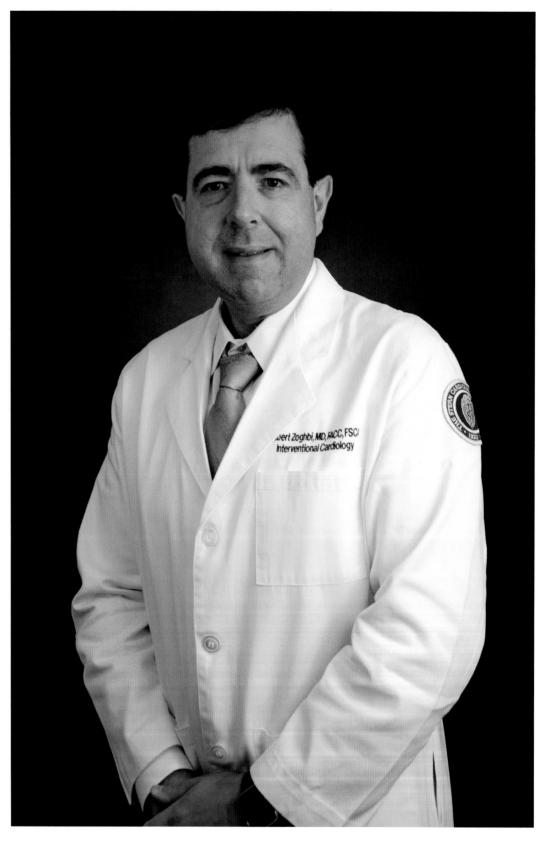

▲ Dr. Gilbert Zoghbi

Photo by Stephanie Norwood

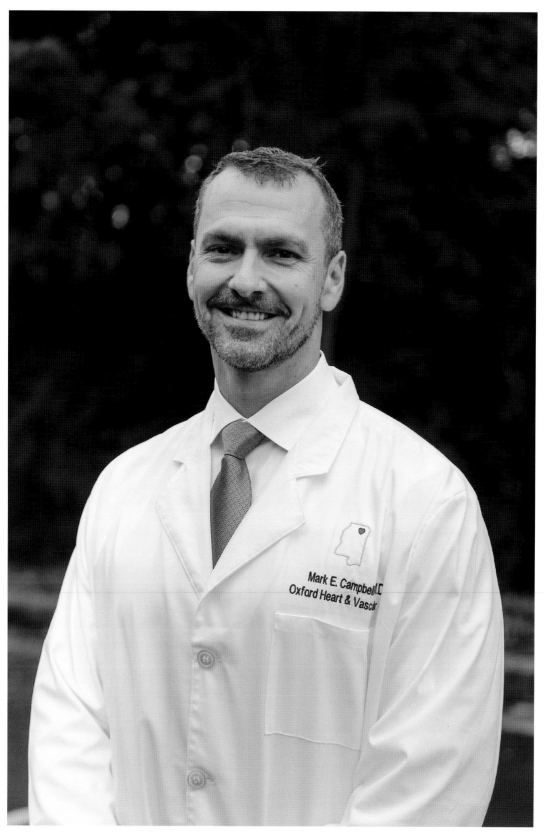

▲ Dr. Mark E. Campbell
Photo by Stephanie Norwood

► Amber Chittick FNP

Photo credit: Stern Cardiovascular Foundation

►► Bob Pegram FNP

Photo credit: Stern Cardiovascular Foundation

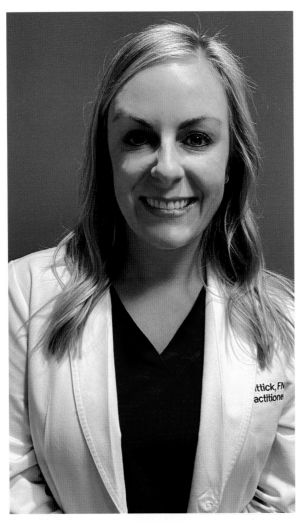

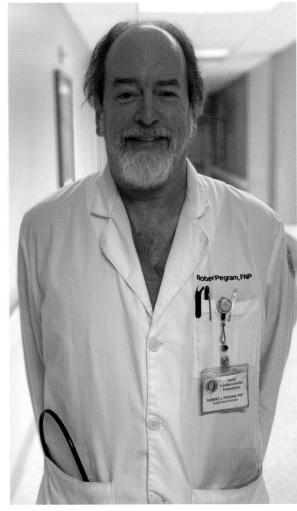

► Jackie Correro FNP

Photo by Stephanie Norwood

►► Ailyssin Dacus FNP

Photo credit: Stern Cardiovascular Foundation

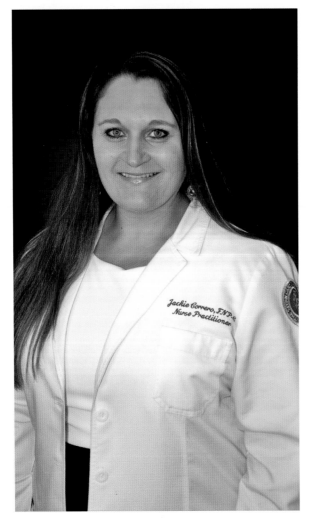

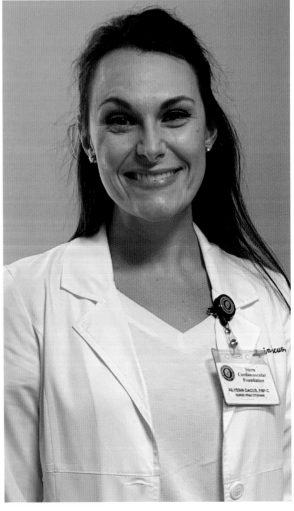

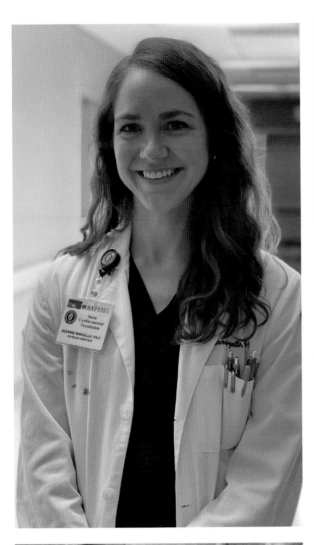

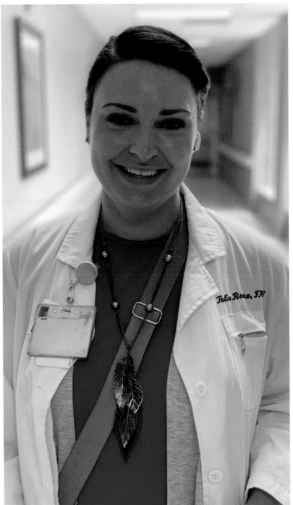

◀◀ Suzanne Margello FNP

photo credit Stern Cardiovascular
Foundation

◀ Talia Reece FNP

photo credit Stern Cardiovascular
Foundation

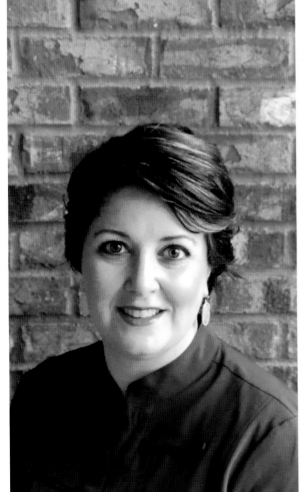

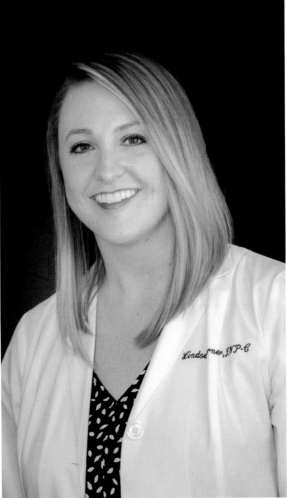

◀◀ Tiffany Leister, FNP

photo credit Stern Cardiovascular
Foundation

◀ Lindsay Garner FNP

Photo by Stephanie Norwood

▶ Raquel Vaughn FNP
   Photo by Stephanie Norwood

▶▶ Lindsey Tartera FNP
   Photo by Stephanie Norwood

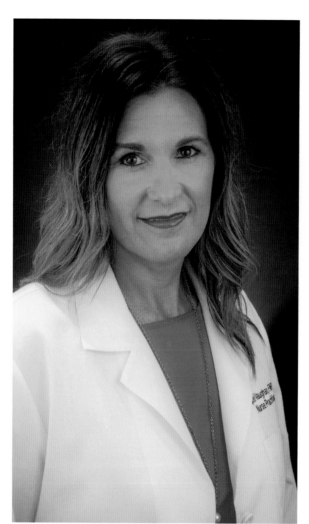
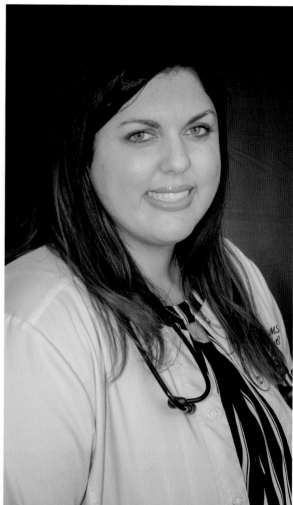

▶ Christy Thornhill FNP
   Photo by Stephanie Norwood

▶▶ Yim Tackett FNP
   Photo by Stephanie Norwood

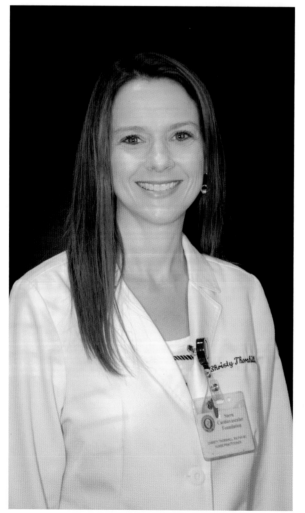
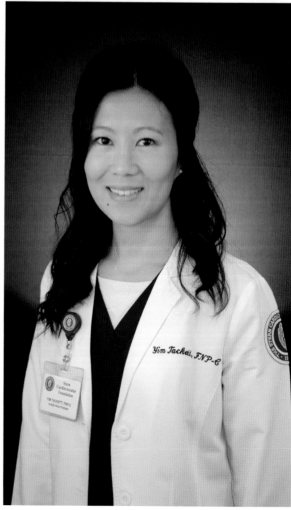

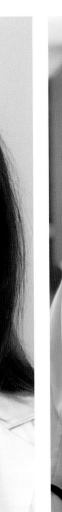

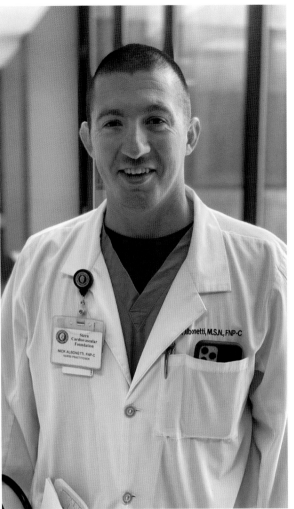

◀ Nick Albonetti FNP

Photo credit Stern Cardiovascular
Foundation

◀◀ Melissa Barnes, MSN,
FNP-C, AGACNP-BC

Photo credit Stern Cardiovascular

Foundation

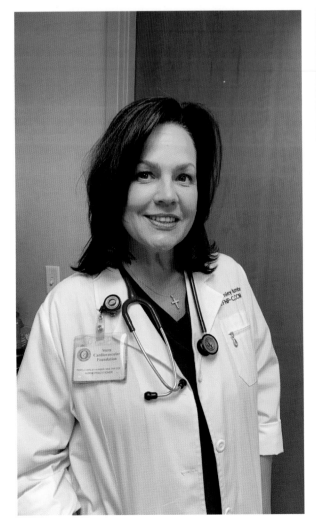

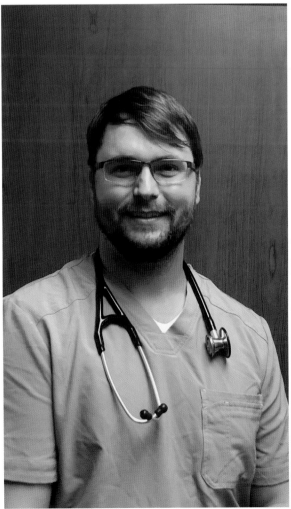

◀ Randall Williams PA

Photo credit Stern Cardiovascular
Foundation

◀◀ Pamela Denley-Humber
FNP

Photo credit Stern Cardiovascular

Foundation

▶ Alicia York FNP

Photo by Stephanie Norwood

▶▶ Elizabeth Zacher FNP

Photo by Stephanie Norwood

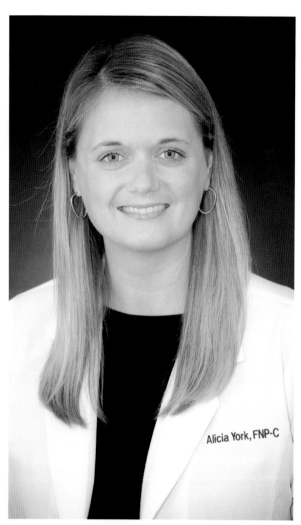

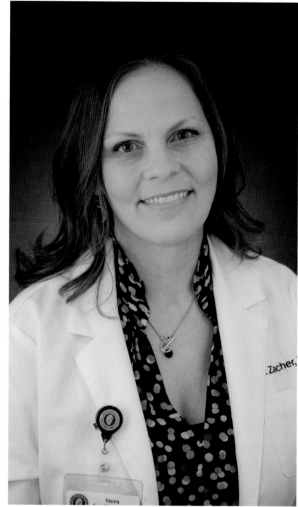

▶ Marissa Austin FNP

Photo credit Stern Cardiovascular
Foundation

▶▶ Kelly Nazary FNP

Photo credit Stern Cardiovascular
Foundation

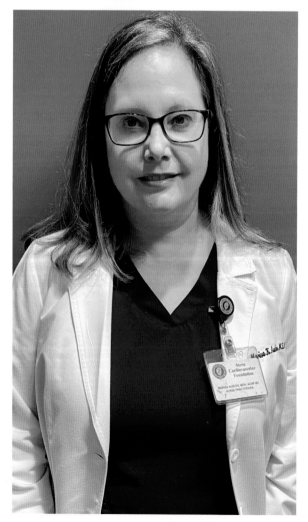

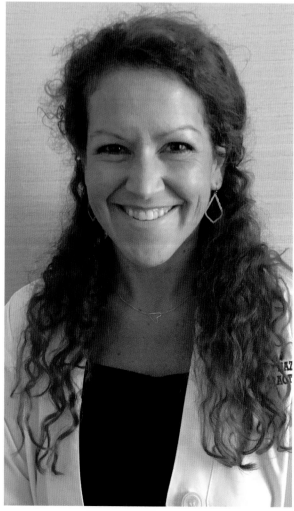

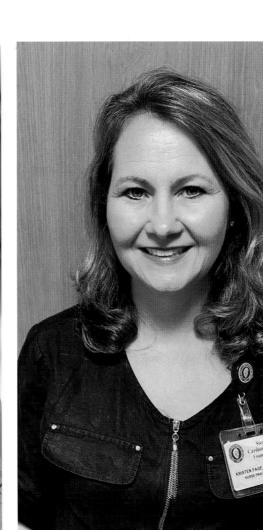

◀ Kristen Page FNP

Photo credit Stern Cardiovascular
Foundation

◀◀ Kimberly Cohen-Greenberg
FNP

Photo credit Stern Cardiovascular

Foundation

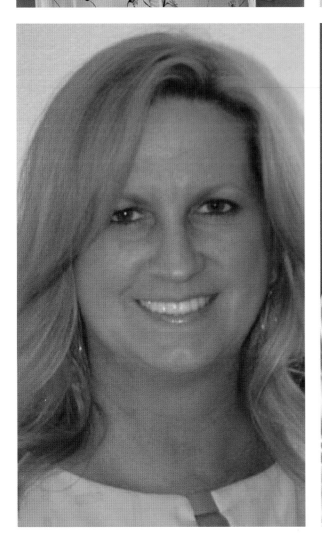

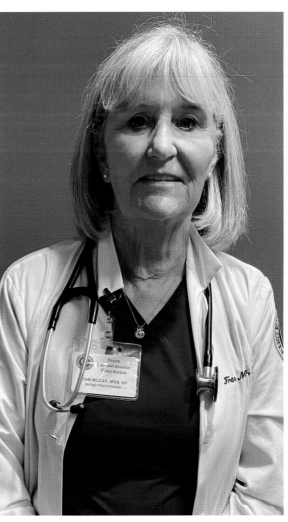

◀ Fran McCay FNP
Photo credit Stern Cardiovascular
Foundation

◀◀ Lisa Reid FNP

Photo credit Stern Cardiovascular

Foundation

▶ Tish Redden FNP

Photo by Stephanie Norwood

▶▶ Hope Ross FNP

Photo by Stephanie Norwood

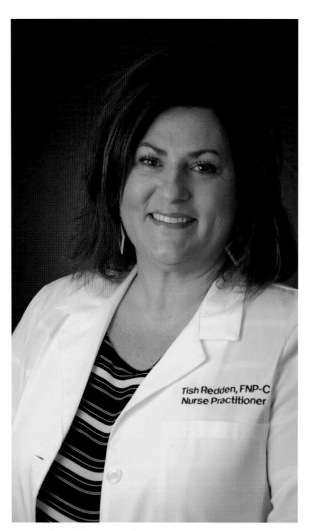

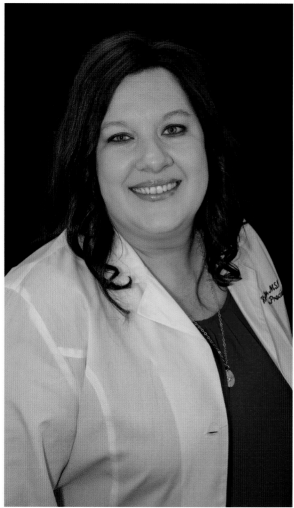

▶ Cathryn Smith FNP

Photo by Stephanie Norwood

▶▶ Jena Willis FNP

Photo credit Stern Cardiovascular
Foundation

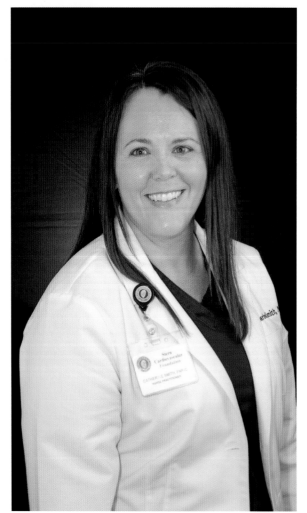

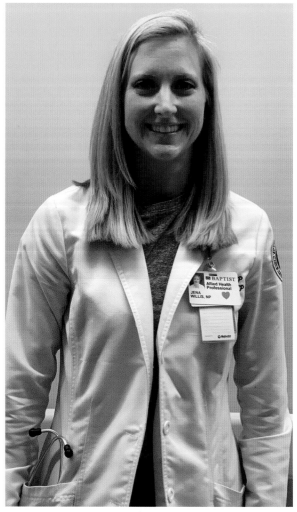

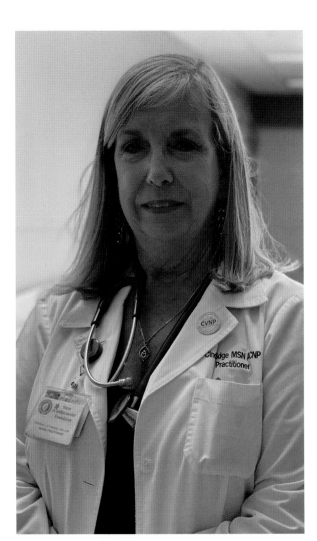

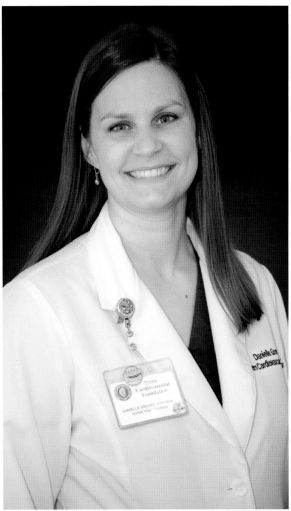

◀ Danielle Groves FNP
Photo by Stephanie Norwood

◀◀ Cynthia Etheridge FNP
Photo credit: Stern Cardiovascular
Foundation

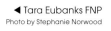

◀ Tara Eubanks FNP
Photo by Stephanie Norwood

◀◀ Brandi Rose FNP
Photo credit: Stern Cardiovascular
Foundation

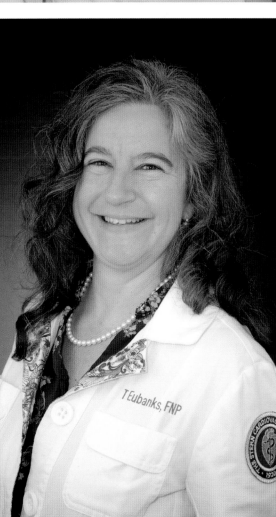

▶ Nalisha Webb FNP

Photo by Stephanie Norwood

▶▶ McKenzie Williamson FNP

Photo by Stephanie Norwood

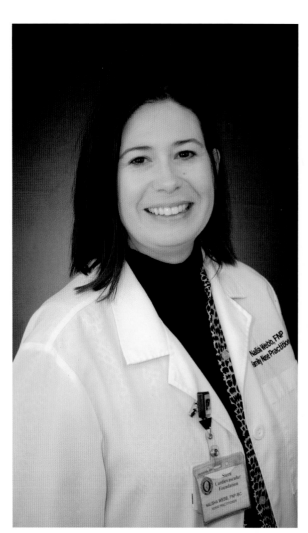

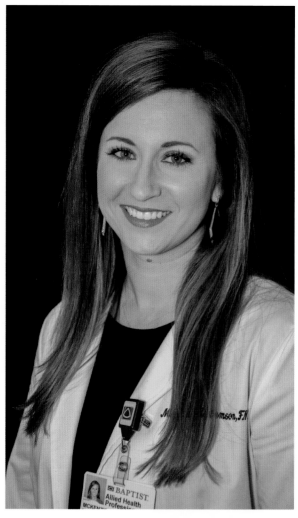

▶ Mary Polly Allen FNP

Photo credit Stern Cardiovascular
Foundation

▶▶ Mayan Kauai FNP

Photo credit Stern Cardiovascular
Foundation

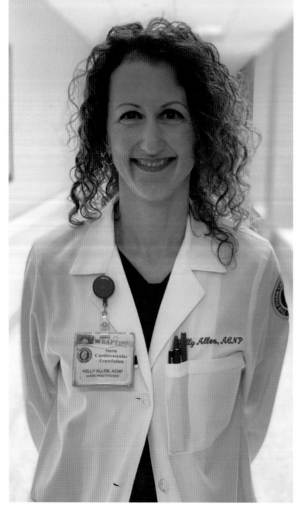

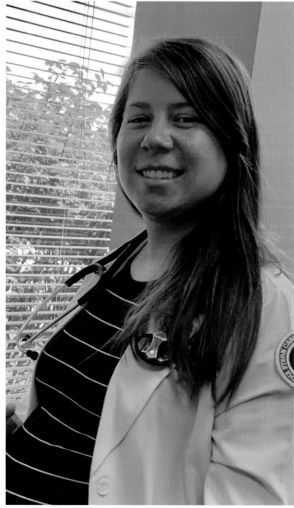

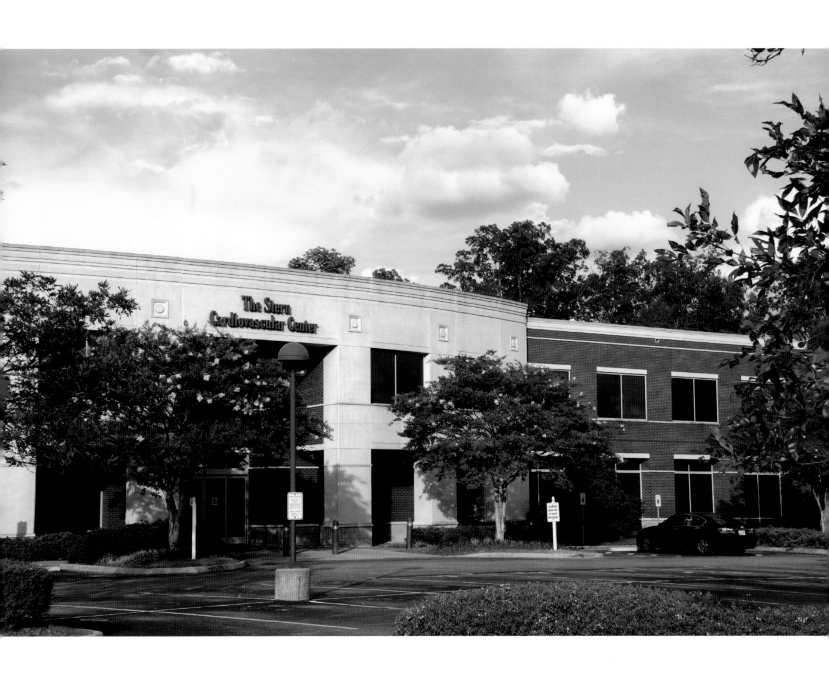

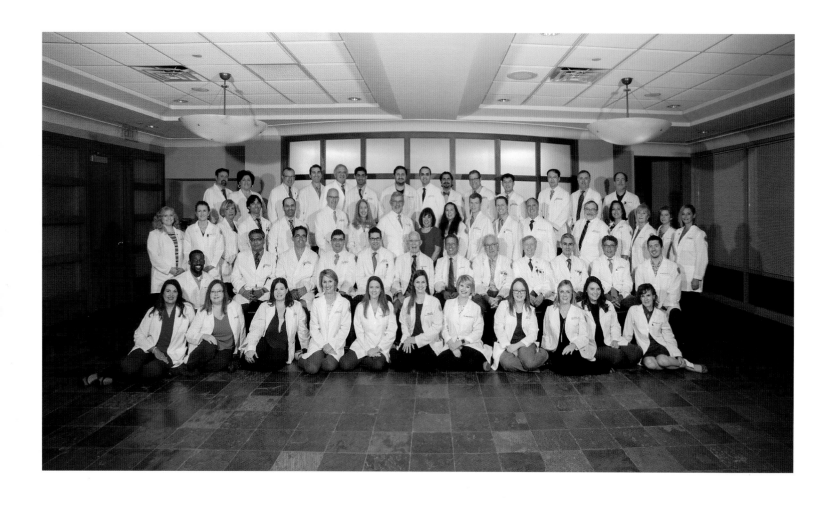

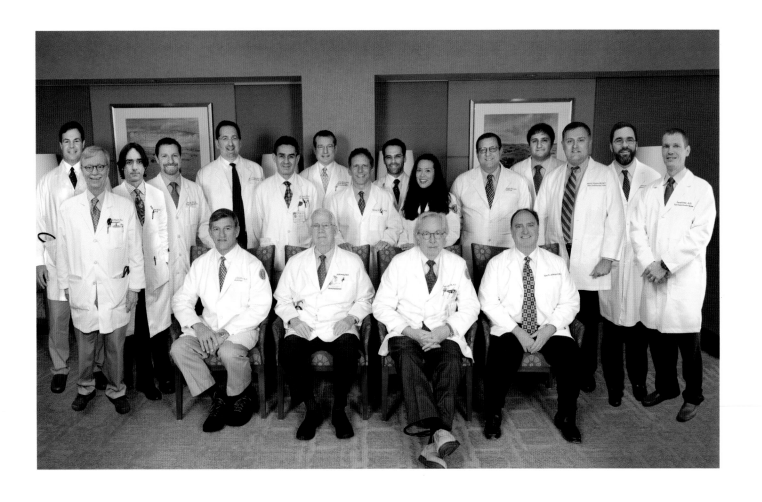

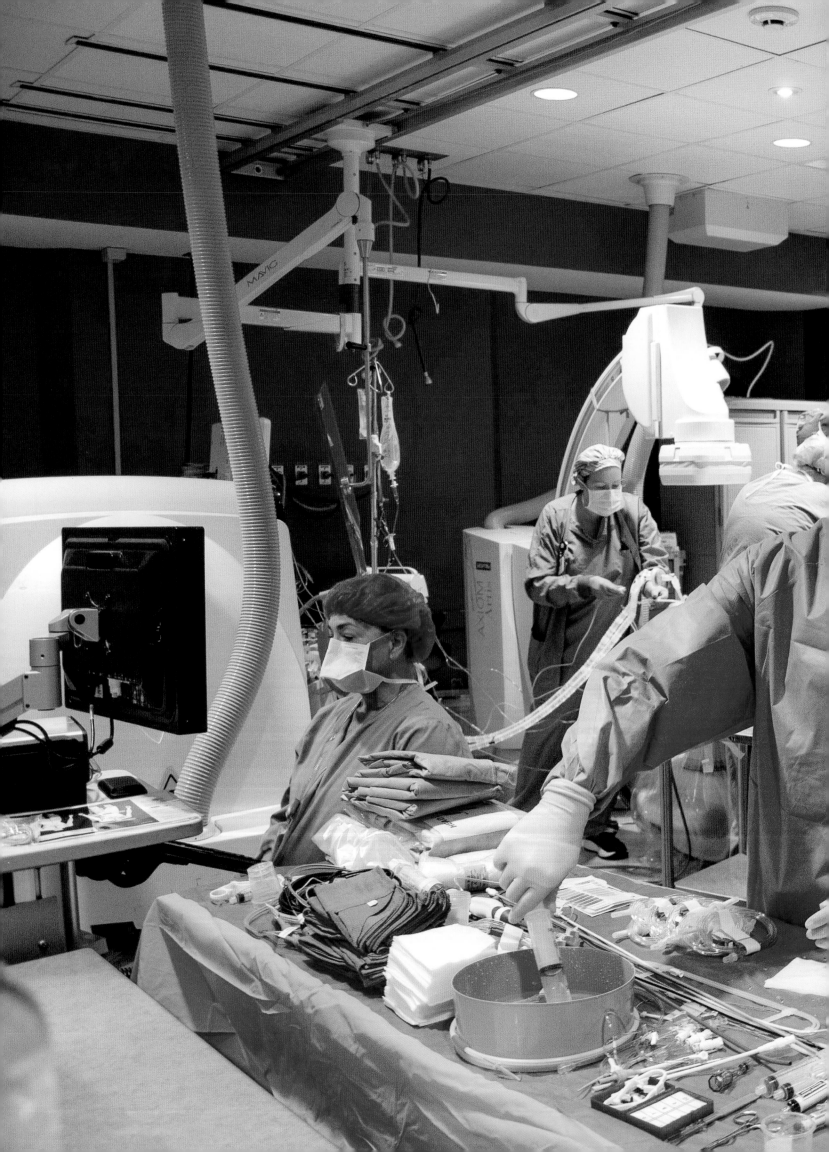

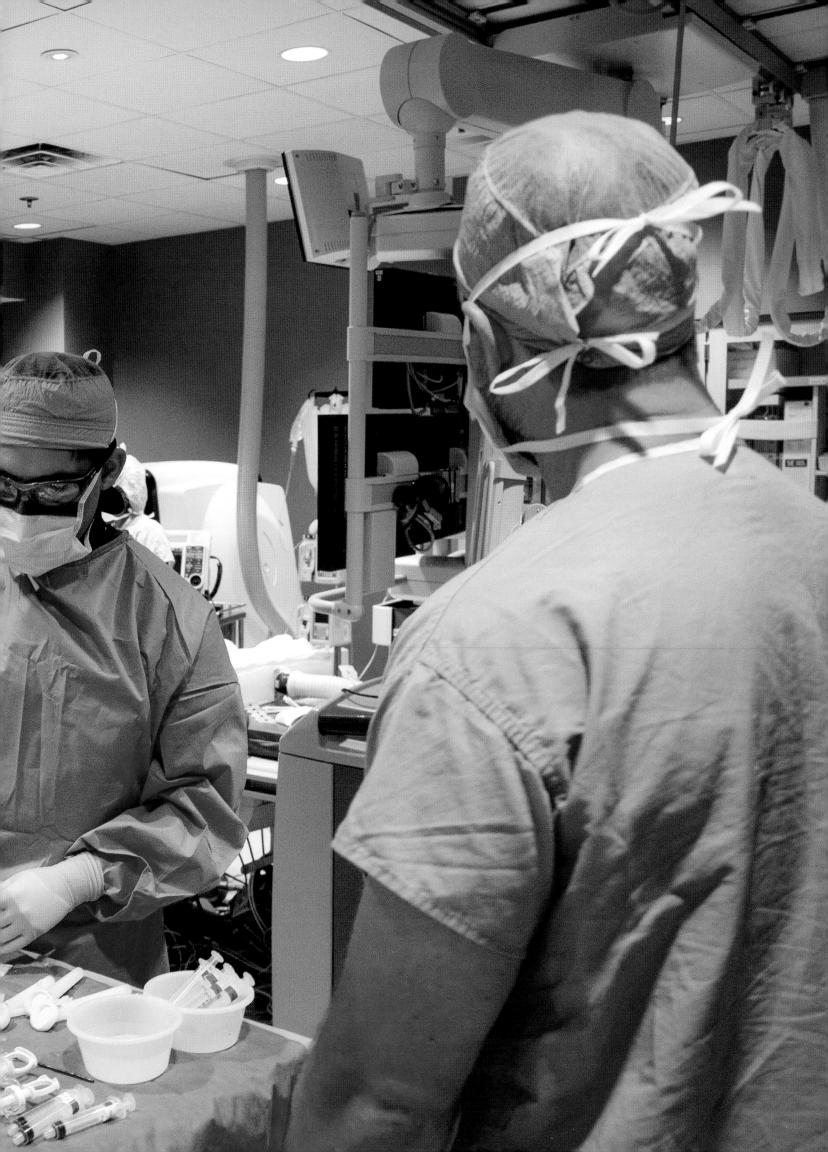

Sources

AMA History. (n.d.). Retrieved from https://www.ama-assn.org/about/ama-history/ama-history

André F. Cournand – Biographical. NobelPrize.org. Nobel Media AB 2019. https://www.nobelprize.org/prizes/medicine/1956/cournand/biographical/

Atherton, Jim. (2011). Development of the Electronic Health Record. Virtual Mentor, 13(3): 186-189. doi: 10.1001/virtualmentor.2011.13.3.mhst1-1103

Besterman, Edwin, and Creese, Richard. (1979). Waller—Pioneer of Electrocardiography. British Heart Journal, 42(61-64). https://heart.bmj.com/content/heartjnl/42/1/61.full.pdf

Certification by the American Board of Internal Medicine (ABIM). (n.d.). Retrieved from https://www.abim.org/about/mission.aspx

"Dr. D. A. Brody, A Pioneer in Heart Research, Dies." The New York Times 2 October 1976: 41.

History of the Houston Methodist DeBakey Heart & Vascular Center. (n.d.). Retrieved from https://www.houstonmethodist.org/heart-vascular/locations/debakey-heart-vascular-center/about-us/

History of UTHSC Cardiovascular Medicine. (2019, July 11). Retrieved from https://www.uthsc.edu/cardiology/history.php

Isaac Starr and the Rise and Fall of the Ballistocardiograph. (2018, February 16). Retrieved from https://www.pennmedicine.org/news/news-blog/2018/february/isaac-starr-and-the-rise-and-fall-of-the-ballistocardiograph

Kalin, Berkley. (1968). An oral history with Dr. Berkley Kalin/Interviewer: Neuton Stern, Beatrice Stern. Oral History of the Memphis Jewish Community, Memphis State University, Memphis.

Lewis, Selma. "Dr. and Mrs. Neuton Stern: Pioneer in Medicine, Legacy of Community Service, Each in their Own Way Made Things Happen." Southern Jewish Heritage Spring 1998.

Loop, Floyd D. (1987). F. Mason Sones Jr., M.D. (1918-1985). Annals of Thoracic Surgery, 43(2). https://www.annalsthoracicsurgery.org/article/S0003-4975(10)60411-0/pdf

Maki, Aisling. (2012, January 9). A Century of Health Care. The Daily News. Retrieved from https://www.memphisdailynews.com/news/2012/jan/9/a-century-of-health-care/

Maki, Aisling. (2012, February 23). Memphis Heart Clinic, Stern Cardiovascular Merge. The Daily News. Retrieved from https://www.memphisdailynews.com/news/2012/feb/23/memphis-heart-clinic-stern-cardiovascular-merge/

Maki, Aisling. (2012, June 4). Medical Realignment. The Daily News. Retrieved from https://www.memphisdailynews.com/news/2012/jun/4/medical-realignment/print

McFarland, Patricia L., & Pitts, Mary Ellen. (2011). Memphis Medicine: A History of Science and Service. Legacy.

Owen, Regina. (2003). Pacer/Arrhythmia Clinic Improves Patient Satisfaction. EP Lab Digest, 3(10). https://www.eplabdigest.com/article/2126

Powers, Mary. "Stern Always Knew He's Treat Diseases of the Heart." The Commercial Appeal 21 February 1993: C3.

Public Health and Promoting Interoperability Programs (formerly, known as Electronic Health Records Meaningful Use). (2017, January 18). Retrieved from https://www.cdc.gov/ehrmeaningfuluse/introduction.html

Stern, David T. (2018, December 20). Family Ties: Three Generations of Board Certified Physicians. [Web log post]. Retrieved from http://blog.abim.org/family-ties-three-generations-of-board-certified-physicians/

Stern, Thomas N. (n.d.). "Memphis Cardiology in Retrospect."

Stewart, Marcus J., Black, William T., & Hicks, Mildred (Eds.) (1971). History of Medicine in Memphis. Memphis and Shelby County Medical Society.

The Electric Light System. (2015, February 26). Retrieved from https://www.nps.gov/edis/learn/kidsyouth/the-electric-light-system-phonograph-motion-pictures.htm

The First Balloon Angioplasty Procedure on a Coronary Artery. (2019). Retrieved from https://med.emory.edu/gamechangers/researchers/gruentzig/bio.html

The Nobel Prize in Physiology or Medicine 1985. NobelPrize.org. Nobel Media AB 2019. https://www.nobelprize.org/prizes/medicine/1985/summary/

What is TAVR? (2016, October 31). Retrieved from https://www.heart.org/en/health-topics/heart-valve-problems-and-disease/understanding-your-heart-valve-treatment-options/what-is-tavr

Willem Einthoven – Biographical. NobelPrize.org. Nobel Media AB 2019. https://www.nobelprize.org/prizes/medicine/1924/einthoven/biographical/

World War I. (n.d.). Retrieved from https://sill-www.army.mil/History/_wars/ww1.htm

A Note from the Author, Samantha Crespo:

Want to know what I love most about writing? Interviewing people. Collectively, the interviews conducted for this project have the power to piece together history, to paint a picture of a time both fundamental and fading. Through these interviews, we can peek into Mildred Pepper Chambers' lab, make house calls with Neuton Stern and take the stairs with Tom. But interviews also bare the human story: the layer just behind the work performed daily by Stern physicians, nurses, executives and support staff. In this realm, employees weep with gratitude for kindnesses quietly bestowed on them by co-workers and patients: Emergency funds raised. Grace given during periods of domestic stress. Funerals attended. When we consider the legacy of the Stern Cardiovascular Foundation, the achievements are obvious. But it's the life-changing, sometimes life-saving, moments personally connecting Stern physicians, staff and patients that make yours such a powerful story. It has been an honor listening to all of you. I especially hope the Drs. Stern would be proud.

The author would like to make the following acknowledgments:

Add Karen, Dr. McGrew's asst.	Frank McGrew, M.D.	Nancy Hardin
Amit Malhotra, M.D.	Jack Belz	Nell Lingua
Arie Szatkowski, M.D.	Jackie Fishman	Pam Glover
Arnold E. Perl	Jada Williams	Pamela Burks
Aubrey Efird	James E. Klemis, M.D.	Patty Hatcher
Basil Paulus, M.D.	Jan Turner, M.D.	Pearl Pollow
Becky Conner	Jennie Turner	Randy Meeks
Brent Addington, M.D.	Jennifer Morrow, M.D.	
Cindy White	Jimmy Ogle	Raquel Vaughan
Colleen LaCroix	John Held	Rebecca Fleshman
Cynthia Bicknell	Judy Jackson	Richard J. Baron, M.D.
Dan Caldwell	Kathy Baker Gwinn	Scot Feury
David Holloway, M.D.	Laura Benson	Sharon Goldstein
David Pollow	Leigh Ann Agostinelli	Sharon Harrison
David Stern, M.D.	Mark Agostinelli	Steven Gubin, M.D.
David Wolford	Marty Grusin	Susan Stern Edelman
Debbie Eddlestone	Meagan Bruskewicz	Tim Harrison
Deborah Ballard	Melissa Reaves	Todd Edwards
Elissa Fine	Nancy Cummings	

INDEX